Bad

Breath

Stopping the Dreaded Halitosis Dead in Its Tracks

(Halitosis Dental Hygiene Odor Deodorant Stop Sweating Natural Remedies)

Matthew Green

Published By **Bengion Cosalas**

Matthew Green

All Rights Reserved

*Bad Breath: Stopping the Dreaded Halitosis Dead
in Its Tracks (Halitosis Dental Hygiene Odor
Deodorant Stop Sweating Natural Remedies)*

ISBN   978-1-990373-94-7

No part of this guidebook shall be reproduced in any form without permission in writing from the publisher except in the case of brief quotations embodied in critical articles or reviews.

Legal & Disclaimer

The information contained in this book is not designed to replace or take the place of any form of medicine or professional medical advice. The information in this book has been provided for educational & entertainment purposes only.

The information contained in this book has been compiled from sources deemed reliable, and it is accurate to the best of the Author's knowledge; however, the Author cannot guarantee its accuracy and validity and cannot be held liable for any errors or omissions. Changes are periodically made to this book. You must consult your doctor or get professional medical advice before using any of the suggested remedies, techniques, or information in this book.

Table Of Contents

Chapter 1: What Is Bad Breath?

Over 90 million individuals suffering simply from bad breath, or have more serious issues with Halitosis. Most people find that the reason for their bad breath is likely to be a result of their mouth the gums, tongue, and mouth. The unpleasant odor is derived due to the presence of bacteria in your mouth caused by food particles that are left inside the mouth following a meal. Dental hygiene issues can contribute to the development in bad breath. The mouth is prone to decay and result in a sulphur compound that creates a foul odor.

If you're experiencing bad breath then you should review your dental hygiene routine. If you are brushing your teeth, ensure that you scrub your tongue, inner cheeks as well as the roof of your mouth. Make sure that you get rid of all debris and food particles from your mouth. It is also important to ensure that you brush your teeth in order to get rid of the food particles stuck in between your teeth. You can use a mouthwash to provide an interim solution for your unpleasant breath. However, if your problem persists, ensure that you speak to your dentist and determine the possibility of teeth decay or gum disease.

It can also happen from other causes such as dry mouth due to diabetes infections, liver issues and kidney disease. Smoking cigarettes is a different cause. Most cancer patients find that they suffer from dry mouth after having received radiation therapy. The lack of saliva in the mouth may cause bad breath because food particles aren't washed out. Some other reasons you could have bad breath are diet, stress, old age, hormonal issues, and even snoring.

If you smell emanating from your back mouth, it could be due to post-nasal drip. It occurs when mucus released by your nose is absorbed to the throat. It then becomes stuck in your tongue, and may cause a sour smell.

The most crucial thing is required to maintain the odors of your mouth under control is a sufficient amount of saliva. Saliva helps remove the odor of bacteria as well as food particles which get caught inside the mouth. While you rest, the amount of saliva produced is less. This is the reason that the majority of people awake having a smattering of morning breath. In order to get rid of morning breath, you just need brush or floss your teeth regularly so that the smell is taken off. Consuming breakfast is another method to remove the morning breath because this can stimulate saliva and for all.

Bad Breath Can Damage Your Career

While bad breath may impact your social life, it also can affect the job market and your professional career. If you're hoping to secure the job you would like, you may want to clean your teeth regularly and steer clear from cafe. The reason is that certain studies have shown that those with poor breath are more likly to get jobs than those who have fresh breath.

If you believe that your breath is bad, There are several things you could focus on to get rid of the problem for example:

Careful while brushing your teeth. Be sure to brush your gums, inside of your cheeks and tongue and even the mouth's roof.

Make sure to floss between your teeth at least every day. Make sure that all food particles have been removed out of your mouth as well as the space between your teeth.

• Drink lots of water as well as other fluids to ensure that your mouth stays moist. Saliva can help cleanse your mouth and will provide some relief from bad breath prior to it begins.

Drinking coffee is not recommended; coffee has a distinctive scent within your mouth. It may cause dryness.

• Take time to wash your mouth after each meal you eat, especially after having eaten seafood, meat or dairy items.

Make sure to visit your dentist frequently to check that you aren't suffering from teeth decay or gum issues.

Make use of a tongue cleanser to ensure your tongue is free of the bacteria.

• Chew gum with sugar-free when you're eating, especially when you aren't able to find enough time to brush your teeth immediately.

• Snack on freshly-cut vegetables such as celery and carrots.

Employers are often told that smelly breath is an attractive feature for a potential applicant. Two other undesirable characteristics are body odor, and someone who's unattractive in their attire.

Employers would like to be sure that their employees clean and neat.

The topic of bad breath is an issue that many people shy away from discussing. The most basic thought is "if I don't think about it, I don't have it". It's vital to recognize whether or not you suffer from bad breath, so you are able to take the actions needed to get rid of this issue. If you

Are you scheduled for an interview soon, it's important to be aware of whether you should be focusing on the hygiene of your teeth a less than you normally would. This is particularly true when you're attempting to get a position that requires you to spend lots of time speaking with employees or customers.

How To Determine If You Have Bad Breath

If you are concerned that you're smelling bad, it is important to find out what kind of bad breath you're suffering from in order to determine the best measures to get rid of it. The causes of bad breath fall into three groups:

(1) fresh breath in the morning, (2) temporarily bad breath (3) persistent bad breath (3) pervasive bad breath.

There are a variety of ways to determine whether you've got bad breath, so you can discover a solution:

* If you notice that the gums are bleeding when you floss or brush your teeth, it's sure that you've got bad breath, too.

Examine your gums to determine if they are swelling and red If so look red and swollen, then your breath is bad.

* Sometimes, it is suggested that you identify your bad breath by blowing out your mouth, putting it into a plastic bag, after that, breathing rapidly into the bag with your nose. It is possible to smell of your breath applying this technique, however generally, it doesn't be effective because your nose is already accustomed to the breath scent.

Place your tongue out to the maximum extent you are able. After that, lick your upper arm or the inside of your wrist. For four seconds, you should feel the scent where the licked area was.

Purchase an BreathAlert device at a pharmacy. It is operated by a battery device, and it provides the reading as the four grades ranging between no breath and severe bad breath.

* Place a piece of cloth that is gauzy on your tongue so far as you can, without vomiting. Give it a while. Then, take the gauze out then let it dry, the next time, sniff it.

* If you're an addict, you may are suffering from breath odors of smokers.

• Ask your dentist dental hygiene professional; they are well-adjusted to getting asked this query.

It can result through a myriad of causes starting from food you consume or a medical issue. A dentist is able determine if your smell is the consequence of tooth decay or gum disease. If the bad breath you are experiencing results from dental issues, they should be gone after you've received treatment from your dentist.

Chapter 2: Do You Have Chronic Bad Breath?

A lot of people have problems with persistent bad breath. It is when you are constantly smelling bad that will stop you in your conversations, regardless of the location, whether it's at your job or personal daily. Bad breath that is persistent may be the result of presence of a bacterial oral illness or an illness or condition of some kind. Bad breath that is persistent can have an adverse impression on individuals you interact with from daily. In reality it's vital to know whether you're suffering from persistent bad breath or not. If you believe you're dissing people by your persistently bad breath take a look at the following tips to help you determine whether your breath problems will be a cause for concern or not.

The most simple thing you can do for yourself to determine if you suffer from chronic bad breath is to determine if you are smelling bad within your mouth. It is mostly due to the decomposition of food particles put back into your mouth after eating any kind of food. When you brush your mouth and tongue properly following a meal, you should never have bad breath, and If you do and it goes unchecked, then it causes persistent bad breath. This can be avoided by brushing up your teeth regularly after having your food whether it is breakfast\lunch\dinner\supper. The other thing to be aware of is that if there is an yellow or white coating within your tongue. This could cause chronic bad breath. It can be prevented by scraping it away or brushing it off the tongue regularly. If you let it accumulate over time, there's the possibility of developing bad breath.

The other ways you will be able to determine whether you suffer from chronic bad breath or not is:

If you are standing with the people you love or are close to and they move to you when you begin speaking or offer your a fresh breath gum or a mint for your breath prior to starting to talk with them is a sign you might pick up it could mean that you've got chronically bad breath. If this happens frequently, and you're experiencing a problem, then it's an issue because many people do not come out and mention it. Many people in our lives do not say this out loud and just hint by giving us mints or gum.

In order to prevent chronic bad breath, scrub or brush your mouth and teeth frequently after eating and go to the dentist once the course of time. Achieving a healthy breath will make you more happy in your conversations with your loved and close ones, or in conversation with others. The people who offer the gummint to you and refrain from engaging in conversation.

Bad Breath - What Are The Causes of Bad Breath?

It is likely that you have seen at minimum some people who experienced constant bad breath. It may be due to a bad diet or bad eating habits that results in bad breath, or an illness which is the reason for the problem. Different people experience different reasons of bad breath, and the cause is different from one person to the other. Medical examinations can provide a better understanding of the specific health issue as well as the cause behind bad breath. In addition to dental issues, the cause could be due to the gum condition and throat infections or tonsillitis, too.

The cause is food habits. bad breath

Food choices are likely to cause bad breath, as the mouth is the place where the food particles begin of the canal for food. The smell of food stays in your mouth for an extended period of time and nothing but a thorough brushing of the teeth or gargling is going to eliminate the odor. Certain foods can cause unpleasant odor, such as garlic and onions, as well as tobacco and alcohol also create this bad smell. But, there are foods that help eliminate the smell, like mint or parsley, lettuce, and various other vegetables. Whatever you consume, be sure to wash it well and is not the source of the indigestion. Indigestion can also be a cause for bad breath.

Dental Hygiene is crucial.

The most important factor in getting rid of bad breath is cleanliness of your mouth that you keep. It is essential to brush your teeth every meal, and floss your teeth every day at least. At the end of every meal or eating a snack, make sure you remove all food debris from your mouth as well as the nooks and crevices between your teeth. Whatever food debris that remains there will contribute for an increase in bacteria that cause bad breath. Make sure to ensure that your mouth is free of any food particles. If you don't do this, it could impact your dental health, which could cause decay and worsen, providing more reasons for bad breath.

Visit a doctor

If you've examined every possible cause of bad breath and removed all of them, the final option is to consult a medical professional for a final diagnosis of bad breath. No matter what the reason one should take care of your personal hygiene and keep a clean and healthy lifestyle.

It's enough enough to keep your breath from getting bad in the future.

Halitosis And Bad Personal Habits

It's fairly easy to prevent bad breath. Though it's widely known that mouth smudges are instantly efficient in keeping bad breath, lasting advantages can be derived from small acts of hygiene. The majority of times the occurrence of halitosis occurs as the result of nothing more than a lack of effort or neglect. There may be times when it is not enough to clean your teeth after each dinner when you are dining out of at home, which results in bad breath, especially when your food is spicy. While it isn't ideal brushing your teeth removes the small pieces of food that have accumulated in between your teeth.

The cause of halitosis can be controlled. In time, individuals may be prone to bad hygiene, for instance not flossing or brushing their teeth prior to sleeping or could not drink enough fluids as they need. Infrequent visits to the dentist can also result in the proliferating and growing of bacterial colonies in the gums. They can then become very difficult to completely eliminate. It is possible to find certain bacteria that can be healthy, however those that are harmful need to be controlled. Overall the good hygiene of your personal and regular dental checks is enough to stop the most common causes of the condition from growing.

Metabolic Cause for Halitosis

It is possible for diabetes to be completely unnoticed at the beginning of its course. Studies have revealed that an overwhelming number of people across the globe have diabetes without having ever been aware. The result is a rise of ketones within the blood. Ketones can be described as extremely unpleasant chemicals generated when our body makes use of carbs instead of fat for energy. They are typically excreted out of the body via sweat, urine and exhaled air. Halitosis due to ketones cannot be treated with the dentist on its own. Therefore, dentists might refer a patient to a general doctor even if no causes for oral Halitosis are identified. Also that a higher blood pressure causes a deficit in the immune system. that bacterial and diabetes may be related.

Changes in nature of the food eaten can also cause bad breath. A high protein and fasting and low carbohydrate diet causes ketosis. For those looking to reduce weight or build muscle the body burns more fat to generate energy. This results in the accumulation of ketones in high amounts in blood that later gets to the lung. This is why there are specific diets that are developed by specialists for certain people.

Bad Breath Cause - Common Causes For Bad Breath

The most well-known bad breath

Most individuals, breath odor is an issue when they get up in the morning it's fine after they've scrubbed their teeth and washed their mouths well. As the day progresses, the bad breath might be present all over again, and individuals may avoid the area and not interacting with your.

The smell of a bad meal can be a source of discomfort.

If you've had a meal that was abundantly garnished with garlic, then you'll notice your breath smells like garlic, as well as when you've eaten onions or even smoked cigarettes. Alcohol is also a part of the smell that remains on your breath, making it extremely uncomfortable for people who comes any time.

Another reason that causes the halitosis

The camouflage of bad breath using breath fresheners or sprays for mouth is an effect only temporary and will cover up the bad smell only for a brief period. If the root cause for the bad breath or halitosis cannot be addressed or cured by a professional, nothing will clear the problem permanently. Therefore, you must get right to the source of the issue and then treat that. There could be a problem with your oral hygiene or teeth that require attention and you'll need to see your dentist. If your digestion has been impaired by food you've eaten, you may have a bad smell.

Chapter 3: Bad breath that is persistent

It is possible to find individuals who have excellent dental hygiene and still struggle with the most serious the halitosis. The term "chronic bad breath" refers to the fact that the person is smelling foul emanating from their noses and mouth on a regular basis. Sadly, since these individuals have impeccable oral hygiene, they aren't sure how to take care of this embarrassing issue.

The reason for bad breath

The most frequent cause is bacterial source of the problem that can cause bad breath. It is due to the food particles dumped in the mouth after eating and that the bacterium begins taking in. In order to combat this issue, it is recommended to thoroughly clean the mouth following each meal, and using a good toothbrush can help. The teeth's back is not to be ignored and the brush should be equipped with bristles that go between teeth as well. Therefore, no place is in the dust and all food particles are eliminated.

A proper method to clean your teeth

If you want to be sure you've scrubbed your mouth thoroughly, make sure you take at minimum five minutes and be sure your toothbrush has reached all spaces and corners. If you let any area that are not cleaned, this could create bad breath.

Another point to remember is that not all toothpastes are identical. They can only contribute to the situation instead of alleviating to ease it. Dental products that contain peroxide and baking soda as their ingredients are recommended. The two components will make an enormous difference in bad breath, and will increase your self-confidence in your interactions with other people.

Authoritative Answers For The Common Question: What Causes Bad Breath?

Halitosis, also known as bad breath, is the condition in which a person is smelling bad. The reason for this could come from a number of reasons. For those who suffer from it, it's an unanswerable question why bad breath is a problem in order to prevent it or even control it.

Certain foods can affect the breath.

Some food items have strong odors such as onions or garlic, and they linger in your mouth after eating. Utilizing mouth fresheners as well as regular brushing of teeth might not be enough to eliminate such odors however relief will be short-lived because the smell is released by the mouth regardless of whether the food has been consumed. But, food isn't the sole cause of halitosis however food particles stuck between teeth generally result in bad breath due to the bacteria that live on the particles. Sometimes, a medical issue might be behind the problem.

A few simple ways to treat bad breath

There's no easy and quick condition that can cause bad breath. If it persists, it's recommended to speak with an expert to figure the root of the problem. It is ideal to get an annual dental exam and examine the state of your teeth as well as general dental conditions. In some instances, it is needed to perform test to find out what the root cause behind smelly breath may be. It could be a serious issues in the system, and it's better to get this checked instead of taking matters into one's own control. Whatever the issue, one is able to fix it in a certain degree by maintaining your teeth clean all the time. Poor eating habits or eating habits that are unhealthy can produce bad breath without illnesses or conditions. Therefore, ensure you're eating healthy and balanced meals, so there will be no need for concern about your breath.

Good habits

If there's no major health issue, it's good be a good idea to maintain hygienic practices and stay clear of bad breath. Avoiding smoking is a different way to improve your breath. Simple facts include to clean your teeth following every meal, as well as brush them frequently whether you are kids or adults, and to avoid developing chronic bad breath.

Bad Breath And Acidic Foods

Research has shown that foods with acidic ingredients could cause certain individuals to develop bad breath. If you've tried different techniques to eliminate bad breath and discover that your efforts have not worked it is possible to remove foods that are acidic out of your diet, to determine the results regarding foul-smelling odors.

The process of tackling bad breath usually involves using a number of different remedies until you have found the best one for your needs.

Acids help the bacteria that live in your mouth grow faster. The goal is to neutralize acidity in your mouth to ensure that sulfur compounds are prevented from expanding. One of the easiest ways to do this is to remove certain food items in your eating habits.

Coffee is likely to be among the very first food items you should quit using. Regular coffee as well as decaf coffee are acidic. You can substitute your morning coffee for tea as tea is more acid-free. A different drink to not drink is tomato juice.

Some juices also have high levels acid, which you'll need to remove for a few days to see the extent to which your breath has disappeared or is less noticeable. The juices that are included include the juice of pineapple, orange juice as well as grapefruit juice. Fruits with high acidity should be avoided in order you are able to neutralize the acidity of the acidity of your mouth.

Bad Breath And High Protein Foods

The foods high in protein could make bad breath worse. It is due to the fact that certain food items that contain high levels of protein can cause sulphur substances to increase rapidly. This means for you that your mouth has an environment which is perfect for the growth of bacteria and increase.

Certain food items help in the generation of sulfur compounds than other food items. They fall under the class of "high amino acid and protein foods. Dairy, cheese and various dairy items are on the highest of the list of to foods high in protein that must be avoided. If you're lactose-intolerant, you should definitely stop taking dairy products because the dairy products will remain around longer than you can allow bacteria to thrive in.

Fish is abundant in protein and ought to be completely avoided for the moment to check whether your breath is better. Replace other protein sources like tofu for instance, to make sure you receive the protein you require every daily.

In the case of food items that are acidic, you should beware of coffee until you decide if the smell is caused by what you consume. Coffee, no matter if it's decaf or regular has a lot of acid. These acids help bacteria grow at an accelerated rate. It may cause mouths to have bitter flavor that could cause bad breath.

Chapter 4: Dry Mouth and Bad Breath

If you suffer from dry mouth, it will result in lower levels of saliva. Also, the lack of saliva in your mouth may cause bad breath. The importance of saliva is in health and hygiene of your mouth since it fulfills the following roles:

* Saliva contains the necessary enzymes needed for digestion of food.

* Saliva aids in stabilizing your pH levels within the mouth. These levels effectively control the quantity of acid in your mouth.

* Saliva supplies adequate amounts of oxygen that are required to keep the tissues of your mouth fresh and healthy.

Dry mouth, also known as Xerostomia is when there's less saliva. It means there'll have less oxygen inside the mouth. In the absence of oxygen, an anaerobic atmosphere is made, which is the perfect environment for the creation of bacteria.

The mouth bacteria produce sulphur gas that will make you breath smell bad as well as leave a foul flavor within the mouth.

Your tongue's shape will also tell whether you've got bad breath. The more rough and sloppy your tongue's texture is, the more likely to have bad breath as there will have more grooves where bacteria will be able to be able to hide. Every person has their own unique form and shape of their tongue, which could be an inheritable factor in the breath's freshness.

Certain people possess a swollen tongue. The papillae, or the fibres that line the tongue, are larger than normal. They can also be a trap for bacteria that make foul-smelling sulfurs.

If you scratch your tongue, or rub it with a lot of force to battle bad breath, it is possible to be suffering from "burning tongue syndrome". This condition can occur in the event that you become sensitive to certain situations, such as hot and cold food items. If you've got a tongue that's sensitive, you'll be advised to avoid toothpastes or rinses for your mouth which contain alcohol.

When you recognize the fact that bad breath as well as dry mouth can go hand-in-hand, it is possible to ensure your mouth stays moist by sufficient saliva. Gum chewing throughout the day will help retain saliva, however, make sure you choose sugar-free gum.

You can avoid you from getting tooth decay. It is also a good idea to keep the bottle of water you drink in your bag in all times, so you are able to wet your whistle when you notice that your mouth has become too dry. A bad breath experience can be unpleasant in your existence until you master some techniques to prevent the problem.

Methamphetamine Can Cause Bad Breath

What can you do to determine the likelihood that your child is using the app?

The first and most frequent signs of your child's use of Methamphetamine can be seen in their breath. The breath is odors similar to chemical that is sour and smells. Cleaning your teeth thoroughly and repeatedly won't help to take off the smell. In addition, look over the eyes for indications and the pupils may be diminished. Another indication is dry, cracked lips, bleeding nose due to dry noses, and the symptoms of sinuses because this drug is taken in the form of a snort or smoke.

External signs and symptoms associated with Methamphetamine consumption

When a person is using this drug, he or she is unable to eat and loses weight, which can lead to the stage that they become anorexic. The inability to sleep, excessively nervous or aggressive personality and constant chatter as well as a generally high-energy attitude are the most obvious signs of taking this medication.

One may attempt to eliminate the bad breath with many mouthwashes and breath fresheners, chewing gum, and mouth sprays, but, to no avail and nothing will remove this bad breath caused due to methamphetamine. Whatever is used to conceal the presence of the drug, these symptoms will never be cured. It is important to keep an eye for any changes in behavior in your child. take action to stop the habit of abuse before it's too late for you to aid your child.

Risky side effects from the medication

Alongside bad breath, There are also other potentially life-threatening consequences for health. It is the responsibility of parents to look out for any symptoms and assist your child. The other life-threatening signs are elevated blood pressure as well as a high heart rate, which could turn out fatal if proper care isn't taken from the first place to stop using this medication. The blood vessels in the brain become damaged and a patient could suffer an accident and then be dead.

However, even after the substance is taken off, there are modifications in behavior and symptoms of psychosis within the individual. Parents should be on the lookout for bad breath and then ask the child about what the problem is. The parent should not be afraid to speak up or avoid asking your child questions about this since it will only serve assist your child over the long term. The parent should keep an eye on the development of their child's life to ensure they know the changes taking place in their children's lives at all times.

What to Do About Bad Breath

A person who is sour can frequently an issue. A person in an intimate discussion with another person might feel a sense of resentment when they be aware that someone else has a bad breath. It could also cause the person listening to be prompted to make faces that express the feeling of disgust. They may also feel nauseated and avoid speaking to the person in question for a second time. This kind of reaction is automatic and totally involuntary. The most effective solution to get rid of stinky breath is move out of it as quickly as you can.

The process of dealing with something as stinky breath is an arduous problem. It is crucial that the problem is addressed in a holistic manner no matter if it's something personal or concerns another person, such as a family member, friend or coworker.

HOW ONE CAN DEAL WITH IT ONESELF:

The most effective way to get rid of smelly breath is to take good care of your personal hygiene particularly with regard to dental hygiene and the oral cavity generally. It can help to some degree. Being lazy or not paying attention to the things that affect one's confidence in himself or herself and self-esteem. The result is a slow decline in self-esteem as well. If you are conscious of the smelly breath they have can take advantage of medical treatment similar to the one provided by a dentist in the event that they cannot manage it on their own. The most effective way to eliminate laziness and lack of knowledge is to be aware that ignorance could cause other people suffer too.

HOW TO INFORM OTHERS:

What can you do if you encounter a person who has bad breath? The first thing you think of is notifying the individual. The thing we don't always recognize is that confronting the problem is the most crucial step that needs to be done. The beginning of conversation with a friend may be difficult. The fact is that bad breath could be caused by a health issue and, by notifying that person about the problem, we could protect the person's life from risk in the most extreme of circumstances.

Are you wondering what you can do? One of the easiest ways to start a conversation is to give the person mint or gum and engage them in discussion. A different option is to offer some general remarks about bad breath before offering someone gum or a mint. The majority of people understand the

hint. But, there are some who may require explicit statements about the smell of their breath. These can all be complex and challenging to put into practice however, they are all things that must be carried out regardless.

Chapter 5: Curing Bad Breath

In order to get rid of bad breath, you need know why it is happening. About 80-90 percent of instances of bad breath, the source may be something inside the mouth. It is usually something less serious than having the mouth is dirty. Plaque is among the most common reasons for bad breath. Plaque is a non-visible layer of bacteria found within the mouth. The bacteria can cause bad breath. Additional dental problems like gum disease or cavities may also trigger bad breath. It could result from something found in the gastrointestinal tract or the lung. The systemic infection can also cause bad breath.

Foods that are corrosive can be the main cause of bad breath. In particular, eating a dish with garlic may cause breath that's unpleasant and sour. Others that cause strong breath are curry and onions. They are absorbed within the bloodstream. They are later exhaled by the lung. Tobacco and alcohol are also sources of bad breath. Certain health issues that could cause unpleasant breath for certain people including diabetes and sinus infections.

There are a few things you can take to ensure that you breath fresh and clean as it can be:

Make sure your mouth is clean. Make sure you brush your teeth daily at least twice and floss once a day. The food and bacteria stored in your mouth or between your teeth can create bad breath.

Make sure to clean your tongue. The bacteria that remains on your tongue may cause bad breath.

Beware of dry mouth. Saliva helps keep your mouth healthy as it functions as an natural antibacterial that helps remove food particles in your mouth.

Cleanse your mouth immediately after eating. The water rinse can help get rid of some food particles left inside your mouth following you have eaten. An easy rinse is helpful in fighting bad breath.

* Eat parsley. Though chewing parsley isn't going to help you get rid of your bad breath, but it'll cover up bad breath for a brief amount of time. Spearmint works just the same.

• Fight off plague. Consuming foods that aid in combat plague may aid in fighting bad breath. Foods that can help fight bad breath include cheese, carrots, peanuts and celery.

These tips can help to maintain your breath's sweet smell. If you're seeking a solution that will last, it is important to determine the reason behind the bad breath.

Finding the Right Bad Breath Remedy

There aren't many items in the world more embarrassing than having bad breath. Everyone who suffers from this problem is looking for the one mysterious cure to rid the condition and make their lives more enjoyable. The problem is that the cures aren't all that simple.

If you're among the many people who are looking for answers and cure, where you're most likely to get the cure is an expert in medicine. The doctor can provide you with specific information about which treatment would fit you best. They can assist to choose the best one since they know your body more effectively than others. In the event that you're in need of an immediate cure Here are some options. They may or might not be effective for you, but it's important to seek out the treatment that is the most appropriate for your needs so that any subsequent interactions with people aren't embarrassing and that you're in your own comfort area.

Drink Water!

The cause of the bad breath, which is not due to dental floss or toothbrushing that isn't done properly could be due to dry mouth. If you're not drinking sufficient fluids, it's a reasonable bet that the main reason to your smelly breath is a desire for water in the mouth. Water is essential for good health. bad breath just one of the reasons to ensure you're drinking plenty.

In the event that you find difficult drinking water, you can take a bite of fruit. Fruits contain a lot of water, and they can be a sure way to get more fluids into your body. It is a great method to begin changing your eating habits, that is a second one of the methods mentioned previously.

Change your Diet

Consuming a large amount of meat, instead of vegetables or fruits may also cause bad breath. Avoiding high protein foods and consuming more fresh foods is a good option for people who maintain a regular routine of flossing and brushing their teeth, and drink plenty of water to ensure their mouths are moist and hydrated. They also get enough of fluids needed by their body however, they still have bad breath.

The next time around, avoid the rich steak and opt to eat a nutritious salad. This is one of the uncommon remedies for bad breath which actually works. It is difficult to tell if the remedy is working until you've tested it on your own. Bad breath isn't quite as complicated as most of us believe it to be to get rid of.

Bad Breath Solutions

If you're suffering from bad breath, the first natural remedy which most people consider is to enhance their flossing and brushing habits. But, a balanced eating plan can be a major factor in neutralizing your bad breath. An efficient digestive system effectively can drastically reduce the amount of bacteria present in your body, which is at the root of smells.

Acidophilus is an ingredient which you must ensure there is enough of it within your diet. Research has shown that an imbalance of the bacteria that reside in the intestines may cause the bad breath you have.

An increase in the quantity of acidophilus within your body could be done by consuming the right amount of yogurt, which is high in live-culture.

Vitamin C helps in safeguarding your gums from cell damage and also aid in speeding the healing process. The reason for bad breath is usually due to gums unhealthy. The best sources of Vitamin C are red peppers, cabbage and oranges. Other good sources include strawberries, strawberry, and kiwi fruits.

You can replace any animal protein which you consume with higher fiber-rich foods like fruits and vegetables. Fruits and vegetables can assist to clean your breath since they're high in fiber as well as having high levels of enzymes. In the course of your day, eat fruits and raw vegetables, like apples, pears carrots, parsley bunches. Parsley is an excellent natural breath-freshener since it has chlorophyll. Chlorophyll is the chemical that maintains the greenness of plants and is considered an natural breath freshener.

Consume at least eight glasses of fluids each daily to ensure your mouth stays dry. Also, you'll flush out any bacteria and germs which can build up within your mouth, due to the foodstuffs.

Consult your dentist to make certain that gum disease or tooth decay isn't the main reason for your breath being bad. Be aware that Vitamin C is beneficial for the prevention of gum disease.

Another thing you can try is eating food that is high in fiber to help fight constipation. Research has shown that frequent stool movements can remove contaminants from your body, which may create bad breath. If you consume large quantities of animal products, you will take in a large amount of bacteria that enters the bloodstream, which is then absorbed into the lungs. It is eventually exhaled in the form of bad breath. The best sources of fiber are Peas, brown rice dried beans, figs fruit, wheat products and prunes.

Consuming a healthy and balanced diet can be a great option to ensure the body you are in top shape and performing exactly as it should. The simple act of eating a balanced diet can assist you remove your breath problems.

How To Cure Bad Breath

Bad breath is caused by a variety of reasons.

The cause of bad breath is typically due to bacteria created in the mouth and is fed by food particles left behind between your teeth after having eaten. One of the best ways to make sure the cleanliness of your mouth healthy after eating is to clean your teeth. You should make sure to do it after each meal in order to stop the buildup of bacteria. So, you'll avoid having bad breath.

Food particles that are stuck to the dental cavity allows bacteria to multiply and can make the problem worse in the event that it is not dealt with quickly. This is more prevalent with vegetarians and meat eaters, than with people who are vegetarians exclusively. The bacteria are attracted by the food particles that are left inside the mouth between teeth, after eating.

Chapter 6: Visit the dentist

If none or none of these is assisting you get rid of bad breath, then it's definitely the time to visit the dentist. Your dentist may perform thorough cleaning of your mouth as well as determine whether there's any other root cause behind the bad breath. Find out how you can maintain your mouth in the same manner that it did after an expert cleaning. Learn how to care for it just in the same manner for the rest of your life.

The Main Cure for Bad Breath

Have you ever wondered why you aren't always able to get people's attention from your conversations with them? It could be due to you haven't found an effective remedy to bad breath. It is possible that you're one of those suffering from bad breath or halitosis, and are finding it difficult to find a remedy to stop bad breath. If foul-smelling breath has been causing you to think about it It's the time to find a solution to bad breath.

BACTERIA -THE REASON FOR HALITOSIS:

The majority of instances of halitosis can be traced to the bacteria within the mouth. A majority of them remain in the mouth behind the tongue. Therefore, to eliminate bad breath, one will be required to remove the bacteria that cause bad breath from their homes inside the mouth and around places.

Bacteria are able to multiply in alarming speed anyplace in your mouth whether in the nooks between your teeth, or in your tongue. The reason for this is food passing in the mouth. Food particles are often able to stay in your mouth following eating, particularly between your gum line or between the teeth and then the bacteria grow out of the mouth. The bad breath that is caused by bacteria typically originates from this.

DISLODGING THE BACTERIA - HOW?

Brushing regularly is the best method to eliminate harmful bacteria out of your gums and mouth. A cure of bad breath usually involves regular brushing at least 3 times per daily and brushing your tongue regularly as well. The texture of your tongue is a favorite home of the bacteria that cause halitosis. A common practice we use as a remedy for bad breath is to make use of gum or mouthwash and it only leads to the concealing of the smell, and, in the absence of gum or mint it remains bad. In contrast cleaning your teeth and flossing can result in the permanent removal of bad breath-causing bacteria.

Neglecting your bad breath simply using gum or mints could be a bad idea. regular flossing and brushing may be the sole remedy of bad breath. If it appears difficult to manage it is possible to seek out assistance from a professional such as dental professionals.

The most effective solution for bad breath is really a refreshing sensation. The removal of halitosis with proper and regular treatment of your oral hygiene will allow you to speak confidently. There is a saying that about one in four people have bad breath. It is important to remove it, if you don't wish to become that person.

Bad Breath Remedies For Home Use

The problem of bad breath can become the social issue of any person suffering from it. It is difficult to interact with others without feeling uncomfortable and always conscious of their shortcomings. Many people can't afford going to the doctor and others do not want to go, particularly for dentists. If you fall into this category, there are remedies at home that may be able to help but they won't necessarily cure the issue, but making it less noticeable to a certain extent.

Clean and thorough habits for cleaning

Maintaining good oral hygiene and having clean teeth is the best way to prevent. It is therefore important to clean your teeth at the end of each meal, and floss every day at a minimum. If you are unable to do the simplest thing, then this indicates that you or are not aware of the issue, or you aren't concerned about maintaining good dental hygiene. It is the initial step to help you eliminate unpleasant breath.

Eating avocado helps bad breath

The fact is that it's not an widely well-known fact, however, eating avocado may reduce bad breath by a significant amount. Naturally, you shouldn't take the risk of overeating too. It is readily available at every supermarket and can help in tackling bad breath to a large degree.

Cut down on your protein consumption

If you're conscious of having bad breath, then determine the cause for the same. You might be eating protein rich foods such as eating too much steak or chicken or meat. The bad breath will definitely increase. Switch to eating greater amounts of fruits and vegetables and observe the improvements of your appearance. Through changing the way you eat, you'll reduce or eliminate bad breath totally.

Drink more water and start drinking it regularly.

A common reason for bad breath is dry mouth. Water intake will not be the only solution, but will also aid in a variety of other health issues as well. It is possible to drink water straight or eat lots of water-based fruits and juices in order to boost the amount of fluid consumed regularly. It is highly recommended that you drink drinking water from a measuring bottle, and then try to drink it all up. So, you'll be aware of the quantity of water taken in and will be able to gradually increase the amount each day.

Herbal Remedies For Bad Breath

There are numerous people who claim that herbs work to treat bad breath. If you have trouble with smelly breath, it might be beneficial to consider trying the herbal remedies listed below to determine if they can help improve the taste of your breath.

* Anise: Anise seeds are the licorice flavor of a seed which will kill bacteria that reside in your mouth, and also disguise the odor. Other seeds worth trying include the dill, fennel, and cardamom.

* Cloves Cloves have been regarded as an effective antiseptic. Create a clove-based mouthwash to apply twice daily. Put 3 cloves whole into 2 cups of water that is boiling. Allow the mixture to steep for approximately 20 minutes. Then, pour the mixture into filter and place the liquid in a Jar.

Lemon: Cut the lemon wedge and place some salt over the stop. Drink your lemon until all the juices go away. This can help get rid of bad breath after you've consumed garlic or onions.

* Parsley: You can chew on the parsley leaves for a couple of minutes. Parsley is used over the years for the development of fresh and pleasant breath. Mint is just as effective as parsley.

* Fennel is a great option for fighting bad breath. There are two ways to utilize fennel in fighting unpleasant breath. (1) to

chew on the leaves in a slow manner in order to create saliva inside your mouth. Or (2) you can take the capsule of fennel (found in the health food store) and then open it by mixing its components with baking soda to ensure that you get the paste. Make use of this paste for brushing your gums, teeth and your tongue.

Folk Remedies for Bad Breath

Through the years, there's been numerous traditional remedies for tackling bad breath. The effectiveness of these remedies will depend on you. One of the most used traditional remedies for treating ailments is to make consumption of vinegar made from apple. Every meal, take one teaspoon in apple cider vinegar, either by itself or in an ice-cold glass. It will not only help combat bad breath, but it can help you digest your food.

Make sure to brush your teeth with baking soda to help reduce or completely eliminate bad breath. Baking soda can help neutralize acids that are present that are present in your mouth. This can encourage the development of bacterial. Also, you can look for dental pastes composed of hydrogen peroxide in order to get the same result.

The peroxide in hydrogen is also beneficial for keeping your sinuses clean. A sinus infection can cause your breath to become foul that can be very uncomfortable. Mix hydrogen peroxide (sold in pharmacies with the strength of 3 percent) by about 50 percent water. Put about 5 to 10 drops in every nostril. Be sure you breathe deeply.

Gargling your mouth with salt water is another method that will flush out any oral bacteria. Also, you'll be washing to eliminate mucus and food particles which could cause bad breath. Be sure to gargle deeply back into your throat to ensure that your tonsils are flushed.

A Simple Cure for Bad Breath With Zantac

The root cause of the smell will aid in eradicating the issue and it is important to identify the root issue that causes this. Acidity-related digestive problems could cause bad breath. the use of antacids will assist in getting rid of the smell of bad breath.

Chapter 7: How can Zantac help with bad breath?

Zantac assists in eliminating the acidity that is present in the stomach, which can cause the ulcer. This helps to reduce the amount of heartburn and acid reflux are reduced. It will also eliminate the smells emanating out of these gasses that are leaking from the stomach. Alongside Zantac the antibiotic can be prescribed for treating stomach bacteria as well as the ulcer. go away. By combining this treatment, this issue, bad breath will also be treated. It is important to identify the source of bad breath, and address the issue instead of relying on external remedies.

See a physician for the cause

If someone has a ongoing health issues, it is advised to consult with their physician to find out the root cause behind the issue. Also, if someone has an unpleasant breath, which is coupled with burning in the chest and other digestive issues such as vomiting and nausea, it's best not to attempt at-home remedies, but seek an expert opinion. A doctor may need several tests to identify the cause of bad breath and burning of the heart. If the diagnosis is found as a digestive issue then Zantac is a great remedy quickly.

Although Zantac is available from a pharmacy, it has different strengths. It is recommended to talk with a doctor prior to purchasing it to yourself. But, if you think there's the possibility of a delay when you visit the doctor, it is possible to begin taking the drug while waiting for the decision.

How to Cure British Columbia Bad Breath

If you live within British Columbia or in Timbuktu the issue of bad breath can be an issue. The effects of bad breath can affect numerous aspects of our lives including the capacity of an individual to find a decent job, to make friends and socialize as well as to locate that special person and have a prosperous romance, as well as many others of a similar nature. British Columbia bad breath is just another kind of smelly breath. The most important aspect is the way you handle the issue.

Visit a Specialist

There is no doubt that British Columbia bad breath happens to be quite difficult to get rid of. The majority of the time, it is imperative to consult a physician who is specialized with British Columbia bad breath who has had plenty of experience dealing with it in order in order to successfully treat it. If you're able to get advice from a regular physician or perhaps an intern. However, if you aren't able to do that go to the dentist to determine if they're competent in treating this condition.

Going to see a dental professional to see a dentist in British Columbia bad breath is an excellent way to make sure you are at the top of your game it is possible to be. it is pretty crucial. Dental health and gums are an even greater part of overall well-being than you thought likely.

Alleviate it on Your Own

If you're an resident of British Columbia, remember that the treatment for bad breath in British Columbia is by the same method like elsewhere. Make sure your mouth is clean as it is possible to do by regularly flossing and brushing your teeth to clean the spaces between your teeth every day as well as rinsing your mouth with the antimicrobial mouthwash. In addition to successfully removing British Columbia bad breath, these methods also help ensure healthy health of your teeth and gums that is an essential element of making sure that your body is remain in top form.

Do Not Despair

No matter if you live regardless of whether you are in British Columbia or Timbuktu, be aware that bad breath can be the same treatment as everywhere else. To determine the most effective treatment for your situation, you have be aware of the part that is causing your

Food or lifestyle triggers the bad breath, and once you've identified the cause of the problem, your odds of getting free of bad breath are extremely high.

Leave Bad Breath Treatment To Your Dentist

Fresheners for your mouth make lots of sense. It could be that there is a particularly strong ingredient in your meals you take in your outside environment or perhaps you're fond for onions or garlic. It can be challenging for family members as well as family members to find the courage to let you know that you might suffer from halitosis. However, dentists is not afraid of telling you this. The use of oral fresheners purchased from the store without prescription are not the best solution anyway. The short-term remedy isn't sufficient if the problem is frequent or appears to be not related to eating.

A dentist will need to carefully examine the interior surfaces of your mouth to determine whether you suffer from halitosis before selecting a series of treatment options to address the specific issue. In some instances drinking a lot of fluids, or simply chewing gum may be sufficient to get rid of dry mouth, which is a source of odorless compounds while you breathe out.

Though it's usually children who are responsible for their bad brushing habits Sometimes, even adults are prone to being negligent too. The regular brushing of your tongue and getting rid of any pieces of food that are stuck between the teeth are practices that can significantly minimize the appearance of bad breath. Dental professionals are capable of getting rid of plaque build-up over time. They can also treat gum problems, and suggest antibiotics for treating bad breath.

Treatment of bad breath beyond your Mouth

Dentists aren't able to solve all cases of halitosis on their own. The gum disease could become very sever and necessitate the help by a professional. However, not all cases of bad breath are due to their origins within the mouth. Dental professionals can refer the patient who is with halitosis issues for treatment by a medical professional to aid to treat a common cause. Ketones are smelly compounds that are normally excreted from the urine, perspiration and the breath that is exhaled. If someone suffers from diabetes, not eaten or his consumption of carbohydrates is low ketones levels within the blood increases. Because ketosis could be fatal Halitosis can be a sign of the presence of a more serious health problem. That's why every instance of bad breath that persist for a long time require medical treatment.

The treatment for bad breath can be fairly simple after the root cause has been determined. However, it could recur when the person refuses to comply with the suggestions or modify the lifestyle that led to the issue at the beginning. Since bad breath can occur any time, getting rid of it only means that it won't happen once more. It's recommended to keep someone in your family or a trusted friend who checks your teeth regularly and to never skip an appointment to see your dentist.

Bad Breath - 5 Remedies

In your search for an effective treatment for smelly breath, it is important be able to determine the source of the breath smell to ensure that you can treat it effectively. It is a frequent occurrence, and it's good knowing that an effective treatment exists and that the smell of bad breath can be treated effectively.

The main reasons for bad breath include food dental bacteria, food items and dentures or dentures, smoking. All of these can are responsible for short-term or persistent bad breath.

There is a remedy that is in place for all of these diseases.

1. Bacteria in the Mouth

The most significant cause for bad breath is oral bacterial which can be eliminated by regular and efficient cleaning and flossing your teeth as well as regular scraping of the tongue. Oral bacteria, like their names suggest, reside within the mouth and tongue is among their most popular places of residence. It is essential to eliminate food debris and plaque out your mouth in order to make sure that there are no bacteria inside the mouth. Through the implementation of a routine cleaning and flossing routine dental bacteria as well as the bad breath it causes can be completely eliminated.

2. Bad Breath Caused by Foods

Certain foods like garlic and onions trigger smelly breath, even in the immediate time and the odor is averted through eating food items like cloves, parsley, peppermint, fennel or fennel seeds. It is not possible to disguised because it is a result of it's origins in the digestive system and it is necessary to rest for all day long to get rid of the odor on your own.

3. Bad Breath Caused By Smoking

Smoking cigarettes is the primary cause persistent malodorous breath, as because of nicotine smell, and it puts your gums as well as teeth more susceptible to infection which can lead to bad breath. The most effective way to avoid the possibility of developing bad breath as a result of smoking cigarettes is to stop your habit as fast as you can.

4. Bad Breath and Dentures

Dentures could also contribute to bad breath when they're not maintained properly. Food particles can get stuck inside the dentures. If not taken care of, the food particles can aid in the development of oral bacteria, resulting in bad breath. This is among many reasons you should wash your mouth regularly after eating.

5. Bad Breath Caused By Dry Mouths

The short-term and long-term bad breath may be caused by dry mouths since saliva's moisture assists in maintaining its cleanliness.

If your mouth is dry there is no way for bacteria to be eliminated. Therefore, it's recommended to consume the recommended quantity of fluids each day to wash away oral microbial. In order to prevent bad breath brushing and flossing are mandatory when you have dry mouth.

The only method to get rid of unpleasant breath, is to find the root of your malodorous breath. When you've discovered a solution which can effectively eliminate bad breath, it'll appear like you have a brand fresh start.

7 Tips For Curing Bad Breath

One of the most prevalent ailments in the world of health can be bad breath. The smell of breath can result from a variety of causes. Anaerobic bacterial growth on the tongue could be one of the main causes for this. Proteins in food we eat gets disintegrated by these bacteria, resulting in the production of malodorous gases such as hydrogen sulphide, skatol etc.

Nearly everyone suffers from bad breath once they get up. The problem can be eliminated significantly by keeping a clean mouth. A few people suffer from bad breath even though they maintain proper oral hygiene because of different issues with their mouths or bodies. Certain illnesses can cause bad breath. The exact cause for the smelly breath must be determined and addressed in a manner that is appropriate. The best ways to cure bad breath can be found below.

1. Good Oral Hygiene

The mouth needs to be routinely cleaned to prevent the development of bacteria in the mouth. The consumption of warm water is essential after each meal. It is important to wash your mouth even after eating biscuits, sweets or even cookies. It is recommended to brush twice per day. vital. The common belief is that brushing your teeth in the morning is to enhance your appearance, while brushing at night is to improve the health.

2. Cleaning the Tongue

The bad breath may also be due to yellow or white layer on the tongue. It is most noticeable in the mornings, and must be eliminated twice daily by using tongue cleansers. Be cautious when cleaning your tongue in order to protect the tongue's taste buds.

A tooth pick is tiny pieces of wood or plastic that has a an edge that is sharp. The purpose of it is to remove the food particles trapped between teeth. It's particularly beneficial after eating fish or meat. The use of it must be done cautiously to prevent harm to gums.

3. Gargling

It's very beneficial to wash your mouth with warm, clear water following each meal. For a better effect it is recommended to add salt into the drink. Different types of mouthwashes are offered in the marketplace and. Gargling with mouthwash may also lessen the likelihood that bad breath can cause.

4. Food Habits

The consumption of protein-rich food is as well known to trigger bad breath. In the event that food items like beef such as fish, milk, or eggs are eaten, it's essential to cleanse your mouth thoroughly. Certain foods, such as raw onions have an odor that others might find offensive. According to some, one apple per day could help keep the doctor away but eating an onion every day will keep everyone at bay. Snack items taken, like nuts, taken between meals may also cause bad breath. Following a regular schedule when eating meals is crucial for avoiding bad breath.

5. Drinking Water

Dry mouth creates an ideal habitat for development of bacteria in the mouth. Saliva is vital to keep mouth moist and limit the spread of bacterial. The secretion of saliva is dependent on the quantity of water that is consumed. Therefore, enough drinking water is required in order to maintain saliva production.

6. Mouth Fresheners

The smell of bad breath could be eliminated with the use of natural or synthetic breath fresheners. Primarily, spices are utilized. Chewing spices like cumin seed, clove garlic, ginger, cinnamon as well as others can be beneficial. Citrus fruits can help combat bad breath. Mouth fresheners and chewing gum can be purchased at a store, however caution must be taken during use so as to protect the gums as well as teeth.

7. Proper Brushing Technique

To prevent bad width, a good technique for brushing is essential. The vigorous brushing can lead to damaged gums. The habit of brushing at the end of every meal and snack can result in the losing enamel. The bristles on the brush must be firm yet smooth in order to remove of any particles that are stuck between the teeth. The primary aspect to be considered when brushing is how you're the stroke. The teeth on the lower side must be scrubbed

downwards, and the reverse direction for the upper teeth. The same is true for the surfaces on both sides. The crowns of teeth, reverse and forward movement is advised. It is necessary to do this in both the upper and lower teeth.

If none of the previous techniques work, what else could be tried? Consider the following options:

A. Elimination of the the cause

Bad breath could be caused by illnesses like diabetes, fevers and liver disorders or gastric issues. Eliminating the root cause can remove the smell completely.

B. Modern Medicine

It is possible that bad breath can be brought on due to an infection. Antibiotics as well as anti-fungal and antiviral medicines may help to treat it. If it's due to chronic inflammation or an immune response, steroid are a possibility. Tablets that stimulate saliva production could also aid.

C. Dental Cleaning

An appointment with dental professionals can help lessen the amount of tartar and plaque within the mouth. This can greatly lessen the intensity of bad breath.

D. Filling Caries

Since caries is among the main cause of bad breath it is required to be cleaned with a dental. In the beginning, amalgam made of silver was utilized, however now the use of the use of synthetic materials has replaced it. If the pulp of the tooth is damaged by a root canal, treatment may be required.

E. Tooth Extraction

If the caries are extensive and causes significant tooth damage dental extraction is the ideal option.

F. Tonsillectomy

Tonsillitis sufferers are likely to have bad breath as due to the effusions from the crypts that line the tonsils. These patients notice a significant transformation after a tonsillectomy.

G. Psychological Counseling

The people who suffer from breath problems are often depressed and avoid people with bad breath. It is a self-inflicted loneliness that affects their daily lives. They need to understand that everyone suffers from bad breath. The degree of severity differs. The majority of people manage it through proper sanitation. Everyone has their own distinct smell that other people may be able to find offending. You must ensure that your personal hygiene practices are kept in order to decrease the severity. Support from family as well as friends is crucial.

Many people seek out doctors to treat their bad breath, even if they have no trouble. It is referred to as a the somatisation disorder. People who suffer from this condition typically experience breathing problems, pain and bad breath, abdominal discomfort and so on. If there is any evidence of root cause has to be determined with a proper diagnosis as well as psychological assistance to the patient.

H. Homeopathy

Based on the mental physical, emotional and social health of the individual The medicine used is determined by the person's physical, mental, social and emotional condition. the homeopathic method. Based on the individual's constitution and health, the strength of the drug as well as dosage are determined. Based on the type of coating that is placed on the tongue, its smell or the cause for breath problems and so on. A medicine is chosen based on its appearance, type of tongue coating, the cause for bad breath. In homeopathy, more than 140 remedies are available to treat bad breath, as per the doctor Dr. Robin Murphy. A few of the most common medications employed are arnica, antim as well as sulphur, pulsatilla nuxvomica and psorinum.

Other tinctures that are homeopathic, such as cinnamon Q, kerosot and so on. are commonly used to gargle.

Use Science To Answer The Question "How Do I Cure Bad Breath From A High Protein Diet?"

A majority of those who adhere to the high protein diet tend to strengthen their muscles, or lose weight. These two categories are both faced having a problem with bad breath. They are left wondering what to do about it. One method to rid yourself of the problem is to get consult with a physician and get eliminate the bad breath completely. They both have the challenge of gaining weight and losing weight as fast as they can, therefore they will require expert help to make the best choices regarding their eating routines.

If your food intake isn't in balance, there could be issues

If one is following an fad diet, such as one with high protein, and bad breath is present, it's clear that it is because the food consumed isn't balanced and that you need be able to rectify the issue in order to eliminate the smell. It is possible to lose more fat, but your natural body's physiology also needs to be kept in check.

It is possible to see an increase in the bloodstream of ketones when a person is on an extremely protein-rich diet, which can cause bad breath. The body makes ketones as it uses up fat, if there are no carbohydrates present in the diet. Ketones escape into the sweat, urine and breath. This is the main reason for bad breath in people who have an incredibly protein-rich diet.

What are the best ways to treat people following protein-rich diets bad breath?

The best and only method, and the best method is to include the healthy carbs into the everyday intake of foods. A majority of people believe that the highest amount of protein can only be obtained through meat and seafood but it's not the case. There are numerous vegetarian options which provide a high amount of protein to your diet and also contain some carbs also. A good example is beans that provide an adequate balance of protein as well as carbohydrates, ensuring that the fat stored isn't burnt up in a sloppy way. Another method to avoid bad breath resulting from a high protein diet is to sweat ketones that are trapped within the skin. This can be done by spending a lot of time outside in the sun or saunas, instead of in the breath. Consuming lots of water can also help to flush out ketones from your urine, and dilute the ketones found in the mouth to reduce bad breath.

Chapter 8: Laser Zapping Bad Breath

If you've suffered from a bad breath problem and has suffered from the negative effects it can have on your confidence in yourself can be devastating. Have you sat in the with others and be concerned that your bad breath had an impression? In the majority of people, it is an unfortunate fact that comes with life. Despite the fact that they've attempted my remedies but they are still suffering. The smell of bad breath can be embarrassing or embarrassing when it happens daily.

A major reason for bad breath, and for which there's never previously been a remedy it is due to a type of halitosis which originates from the tonsils. If you're among the individuals whose breath problems is linked to tonsils, it's good to know that laser treatments are the only thing that can give you some relief.

Halitosis that is mild in nature are generally the result of bacteria found in the dental cavities gums or the teeth. The bacteria release gasses that have the smell of bad breath, for example, hydrogen sulfur. To stop this type of breath, clean your teeth on a regular basis, make use of the mouthwash and make sure you visit your dentist frequently for regular teeth cleansing.

Certain food items can cause bad breath for some individuals, especially foods that are strong in taste. Garlic is most likely to be the top cause of bad breath. It can cause a persistent smell that may last for up to a few hours. Other food items that create bad breath include powerful spices, cabbage and even alcohol.

The tonsils could also contribute to the smell of bad breath. It is due to the fact that your tonsils are dotted with pits and grooves that provide ideal for bacteria to flourish in. It is great news that there's now an laser treatment to help make these grooves more secure in the tonsils to ensure that harmful bacteria cannot be able to enter. The whole process will last approximately 15 minutes from start to finish.

The laser helps rid the tonsil of tissue that is infected. This causes the scar tissue forms. Bacteria cannot through this scar tissue, which means they will not have a place to reproduce. A majority of people will be free of bad breath by only one treatment with a laser, while some patients may need to undergo several treatments.

Prior to attempting laser treatment to treat bad breath, it is recommended to test more traditional methods initially. It could be applying mouthwash to your teeth frequently and scraping your tongue. If all else doesn't help, talk to your doctor or dentist to get additional information regarding laser treatment to help with bad breath.

Fighting Bad Breath From A Low Carb Diet

There is a chance that you shed a significant amount of weight while on the low-carb diet, but one result of losing weight is a bad breath. Dental professionals are finding that they are receiving a number of complaints from patients concerning smelly breath. Some patients believe that it may cause tooth decay and is making them have bad breath, but after an examination, dental professionals discover that tooth decay is not an problem. The bad breath that you experience is known as "ketone breath" and has the scent of a sickly sweet. it.

The breath of Ketone is the result from the accumulation of chemicals in the body from a lower carbohydrate diet.

Diets that are low in carbs function because the body uses stored fat for fuel instead of using carbohydrates. If your body fat is used as fuel, smelly ketones, also known as chemicals, build up inside the body. Ketone chemicals then get released into your the urine as well as in your breath.

Thus the bad breath problem is among of the main negative side effects associated with a low carb diet.

A lot of times, bad breath can result from the decomposition of specific food particles which are sulphur-containing. On the tongue, bacteria as well as gums is another cause. Diets high in protein can produce huge amounts of sulfur compounds, particularly in the evening when there is little saliva available to flush away these substances.

There are a couple of things you can try to combat "ketone breath" if you're following a diet that is low in carbs:

• Make sure you take plenty of water to ensure that you can wash off any germs and bacteria that are inside your mouth.

Chew fresh bits of parsley

* Chew gum with sugarless.

• Make the effort to floss your teeth and your tongue each meal.

Make sure you floss following every meal.

You can try bleaching your teeth. The bleaching process can aid in preventing bad breath as it functions as an oxygenating substance that eliminates bacteria and germs.

Breath problems can have an adverse effect on everything you do during the day, from chatting with friends and colleagues, to kissing your lover. If you're trying to shed weight it's not something you'd like to focus on is your breath when you're looking to improve your self-esteem. your self. The

These tips will help you maintain a healthy level of breath, allowing you to concentrate on the weight-loss program you are on.

If your smell persists even after you've been on your low carb diet be sure to consult a physician. A bad breath is an indicator of more serious health issues, such as diabetes.

How To Get Rid Of Bad Breath For Good

The people who have bad breath understand the trouble that it brings, and will do whatever it takes in order to figure out how remove bad breath. It's good to know that it is easy to learn ways to eliminate bad breath, as long as it isn't due to an illness. Simply observe your diet and ensure that your oral hygiene is clean regularly.

What Causes Bad Breath?

Most often, food particles end up getting stuck between your teeth following you eat and gives the appearance of bad breath. The people who eat a diet high in protein typically suffer from this issue. they are forced to wrestle to eliminate bad breath. Contrarily, those who consume plenty of vegetables and fruits don't have any need for getting rid of smelly breath. Fresh vegetables and fruits provide a clean and healthy breath. It's no wonder that we don't see many vegetarians struggling to eliminate bad breath.

Five Simple Ways to Get Rid of Bad Breath

A common person will easily find out how to rid himself of bad breath, if that they are not having a gastric issue or a medical issue. The primary cause of bad breath is the bacteria which feed on foods that stick to the teeth. Use these simple tips that will show you how to remove bad breath.

The first step is to get yourself a great brush and floss. This is the only way to find out how to eliminate bad breath. It is crucial to pay particular focus to your oral hygiene.

Learn to also brush your tongue as well as cleaning your teeth if are looking to eliminate bad breath for good. The bacteria that enjoy feasting on the food that has accumulated in your teeth, also love getting in your tongue. Get rid of them by frequently cleaning your tongue. Then, you're in the process of discovering how to rid yourself of bad breath.

Thirdly, establish a suitable routine for your oral hygiene. The practice can rid you of any bacteria that cause bad breath.

Make sure to brush your teeth every meal and make sure you floss frequently. Using a

The mouthwash disinfectant will eliminate through your mouth all bad bacteria responsible for the smell you have.

Fourthly, stop smoking for reasons of health since it's the most common source of bad breath. If you smoke cigarettes, they creates a bad smell not just to your mouth as well as your clothing as well as your hair. Equipment for dental hygiene such as floss, toothpaste and mouthwash can help reduce bad breath smokers, but they are not able to stop the unpleasant smell that emanates from the body of a smoker. If you're looking to eliminate bad breath, consider stopping smoking.

Fourth, quit drinking alcoholic drinks since they make you smell bad. If you're a frequent drinker, your breath can have the scent of alcohol. No matter what options available and even the use of mints for your mouth, you'll have a hard time eliminating the stink.

Bad Breath In Children

If your child is suffering from bad breath, it's important to determine the root of the issue so it is possible to eliminate the possibility of health issues. A majority of children's bad breath stems from dental decay. When your child's teeth begin to appear, they're at risk of decay. That means you need be practicing good dental hygiene practices starting at an early stage, starting as young as the time of your child's first birthday. Take a toothbrush that is soft and clean your child's mouth when they are nursing or drinking the consumption of a bottle. If you are beginning to introduce foods into your child's diet, make sure that you spend the time to lightly brush to ensure food particles are eliminated from the mouth. Do not allow your child to sleep using a bottle as this is the leading causes of tooth decay.

If your child's teeth aren't the cause for poor breath in your child, there are other issues that could be causing it. Other medical issues could include issues with the throat, sinus infections and obstructions of the adenoids and tonsils. When children are sick, they're more prone to respiratory ailments that can result in bad breath.

Certain food groups could produce bad breath in children. Consider removing foods from groups between two and four weeks and see how your child's breath changes. A few foods to avoid are wheat, dairy and glutens, citrus, oysters eggs, and shellfish.

Bad Breath In Dogs

The problem of bad breath doesn't only affect those which people suffer from. If your pet has bad breath may cause you to feel uncomfortable. A few of the most frequent reasons for dogs' bad breath can be attributed to gum or dental issues. The problem is that the smell of dogs' breath can be the sign of health issues. What you must do is to determine the reason your dog's breath is not pleasant.

The dogs are often affected by an accumulation of tartar on their teeth. After eating, a few particles of food can be left in your dog's mouth. The food particles begin to decay and it's the decay that creates the perfect place for bacteria to thrive. They will also expand to produce plaque. Plaque is composed of minerals, decomposed food items and bacteria. The plaque could affect your dog's dental health and lead the dog to smell bad. Plaque is one of the main causes dental loss in pets because it sticks to the base of teeth, which causes the gums to receding, and then become inflamed.

If your dog's health is affected by plaque you'll see that your dog eats less. At the beginning of the plaque condition, there'll appear to be a yellow or brown layer on the surfaces of the teeth especially on the molars that are large. Dogs with smaller breeds appear to suffer more from plaque than bigger breed dogs. Dental hygiene is crucial for canines to ensure that plaque does not have the chance of forming. It is important to ensure that you provide your pet with an annual dental check-up. It will help save the teeth of your pet and keeping bad breath at bay.

There are other factors that cause dog breath problems, aside from plaque. When your dog is shed the baby teeth, you could discover that your dog drools or smells bad. The bad breath issue is likely to disappear once all the baby teeth are changed by adults' teeth. In this phase of your pet's life, scrub his mouth with the mixture of dilute baking soda as well as water. This can provide your dog with some relief from pain caused by teething and freshens the breath of your dog.

Dogs who are older may suffer from health issues that alter their breath. These include kidney and liver issues. Dogs with kidney and liver issues will appear thin, and will have a very small appetite. A vet is able to tell if your dog's smelly breath is an indication of organ dysfunction. The dog's teeth need to be cleaned, and an antibiotic regimen administered in order to ensure that the bacteria doesn't get into the.

Chapter 9: The Twelve Causes of Bad Breath

Bad breath, which is medically referred to as halitosis can be triggered by a number of factors. Being aware of the causes will aid in eliminating it. These are the most important and common causes for bad breath:

Hyperacidity

Hyperacidity can be described as an extreme acidity in the stomach, or the digestive tract. The stomach has the acid hydrochloric that is essential for digestion. If the stomach is very acidic due to the hunger pangs or gastro esophageal resuscitation disorder (GERD) The smell of acid is absorbed into the lungs. It is exhaled via the mouth and nose. It can result in breath that smells sulfur.

Dry mouth

Dry mouth, sometimes referred to as xerostomia, can cause bad breath due to the absence of liquid that can moisten your mouth. Saliva is the main source of moisture for your mouth. However, in times of stress or anxious and your mouth starts to dry out, it can cause a dryness. Involvement in the salivary glands may also lead to dry mouth. Dry mouth is another cause of bad breath in the morning.

Pulmonary issues

The conditions that trigger a cough, chronic sinus infections, bronchitis as well as pneumonia, bronchiectasis post-nasal drip, as well as other respiratory ailments can lead to bad breath. It is due to the accumulation of mucus the Dittrich's Plugs or pus that are within your respiratory system. The smell is due to the fact that bacteria are present in them. should they not be coughed up, they will cause bad breath.

Visit your doctor when you experience these symptoms that include chronic cough, frequent fever, a runny nose (sore throat), difficulties breath (dyspnea). There are a few situations where people suffer from respiratory issues however they don't show any symptoms. Therefore, it is recommended to get a check-up each year, at a minimum.

Cancer or tumor

A cancerous tumor in your gastrointestinal tract or in your respiratory system may result in unpleasant breath. The cancer causes the death of or putsrefaction of cells, which results in unpleasant-smelling liquids. The result is foul-smelling odors, which can emanate from your breath. There is no way that oral rinses, brushes, or flossing is going to remove this smell in the absence of a tumor is removed or treated.

Metabolic disorder

A metabolic disorder such as diabetes mellitus may cause smell of acetone or fruity breath. It happens when hyperglycemia (too too much sugar) happens throughout the body as the pancreas fails to release enough insulin in order to process carbohydrates. When this happens, the body has to utilize fats for its sources for energy, instead of carbs.

Fats being the primary source of energy is not a normal practice. The process of metabolizing fats to generate energy produces ketones including acetone, the aceto-acetic acid and beta-hydroxybutyric acid. These compounds emit an unpleasant scent that is released from the mouth and nose. If not treated, it may lead to coma, or even death.

Poor oral hygiene

Incorrectly brushing can cause bad breath. Food particles left within your mouth let bacteria grow and create smelly food particles to form. It is important to brush your teeth at least twice each day to eliminate particles of food that have accumulated the spaces between your teeth. If you choose to purchase an oral rinse, make sure you choose an organic brand that will cause dryness in the mouth. Note that dry mouth is a major cause of halitosis.

Medications

Certain medications may cause dryness in the mouth. The medications that trigger dryness and hyperacidity in the mouth can also lead to bad breath, as discussed. If you're taking medication, be aware of the adverse effects associated with this drug, so that you be aware of how to handle the effects. If the medication creates dry mouth, you'll need be sure to drink water frequently. If it triggers hyperacidity then it's best to incorporate it into the meals you eat.

Diet

Food choices can result in bad breath. Hot foods such as onions and garlic can produce an smell that can cause bad breath. The majority of fruits and vegetables neutralize the acidity in the stomach and reduce the chance of breath odor. Chlorophyll is an organic deodorizer that's naturally found in all the vegetables.

Mouth condition

Abscesses of the tooth and gums as well as inflammations cause a pungent odor as a result of the bacteria. The medical term for it is periodontitis, or pyorrhea the abscesses release pus, and also house bacteria. The bacteria always emit odorous odors and can release them via your nose and mouth by exhaling. Scurvy, in addition, is result of a deficiency in vitamin C. Oral thrush is caused due to a yeast disease.

Full stomach

A full stomach can increase the acidity of your body, which may cause unpleasant smells. If you don't have breakfast, you tend to suffer from this issue. Mouths smell regardless of how often they wash it with mouthwash.Don't develop bad breath simply because you're not able to have breakfast.

Substance misuse

Alcohol, tobacco and other drugs can cause halitosis due to of their contents and the method they are metabolized. Alcohol has a fruity scent and tobacco releases nicotine. In addition, the metabolism of substances can produce smells that are unpleasant. The substances that are abused can trigger a range of ailments in your body. These ailments can lead to your body becoming sour and smelly.

One example is that of alcoholism. If you're an addict and you're a result of it, there will be nutritional deficiencies, where the body won't get the necessary vitamins and nutrients. In the event of malnutrition, it will cause smelly body emissions as well as unpleasant breath.

Deficiency of vital vitamins and minerals

Insufficient mineral and vitamins may cause bad breath and body odor. Research has proven studies that a deficiency in vitamin C can cause bad breath as a side result of the disease Scurvy. The condition can also cause bleeding gums, pyorrhoea and an unhealthy oral condition. It is also known as pyorrhea. Inflamed gums and damaged teeth can attract bacteria and lead to bad breath.

Also, a lack of vitamins B12, D, and E could cause problems with digestion, respiration, as well as metabolism. In the event of this the bad breath may occur as a result of constipation, poor removal of metabolites, as well as an accumulation of toxic waste within the blood.

Vital minerals, like magnesium and potassium, as well as calcium and phosphorus are essential to the health of your mouth and body. Insufficiency in these minerals can cause tooth decay, digestive disorders as well as other problems. The conditions can cause bad breath.

Chapter 10: Medical Treatment for Bad Breath

A medical consultation is required when the reason for your breath problems is because of pathological conditions. For this to be determined it is necessary to see your physician for a comprehensive medical exam. The therapeutic drugs, like all other substances, should only be used in cases of no medical contraindications. Only FDA accepted drugs can be taken.

If your smelly breath may be due to underlying medical issues, it is important to talk to your physician first. Based on the physical manifestations as well as laboratory diagnostic tests, a doctor will identify if you are suffering from an illness.

Respiratory illnesses

If you are suffering from one respiratory ailments An antibiotic may be required when the cause is an organism known as a bacterium. Wide-spectrum antibiotics, such as streptomycin and erythromycin, may be administered along with other medications which treat different symptoms like cough, colds, or fever. If your respiratory illness is treated, then you'll be rid of your breath. But remember that you should keep up with proper hygiene practices and a healthy diet. You also need to ensure adequate water intake, adequate sleep and an active life style.

Mouth condition

The conditions of mouth can be easily treated with a proper eating habits and proper oral hygiene. For scurvy cases Vitamin C as well as vitamin D consumption will eliminate the issue because both vitamins help strengthen gums as well as the teeth. For oral thrush, products that fight fungi and ointments like Nystatin are a good option.

If abscess or inflammation can be attributed to bacteria as periodontitis is, the use of a broad-spectrum antibiotic is advised. Examples include amoxicillin anthromycin, cloxacillin or erythromycin and the ones mentioned in respiratory diseases.

Dry mouth caused by acidity

Dry mouth may be result of hyperacidity. So it is necessary to lower the level of your stomach that is acidic with antacids or fundamental solutions that can help neutralize acid within the stomach. Antacids comprise: Maalox, milk of magnesia Mylanta and Kremil-S.

Tumors and cancer

Cancerous tumors can be eliminated, and the treatment for cancer usually is by chemotherapy. As of now, bad breath can be an issue However, it is important to concentrate on remaining healthy while fighting cancer.

Abuse of drugs

It is recommended to address alcohol abuse by working in a team. There are a few medications that available that can induce nausea upon the very first drink However, overcoming addiction should be done by an entire group of people who are with you. Smokers looking to stop smoking for health reasons and improve their life style can receive support from groups However, they must also use nicotine patches or vapors as they transition off from smoking tobacco.

Insufficient minerals and vitamins

An affluent diet will supply the minerals and vitamins that you require on a daily basis, however frequently, the diet we eat is inadequate. In order to fix this issue problem, there are a variety of multivitamins you can consume. Multivitamins can supplement your diet with missing essential nutrients your body requires. The best vitamins without sugar are those that do not contain excessive sugar can be harmful for your body. Be sure that you'ren't in any way allergic to their ingredients.

The treatment is based on to the signs and symptoms. And in the case of severe conditions the advice of your physician is essential to the successful completion of the treatment.

Chapter 11: Natural Methods to Eliminate Halitosis

The best way to get the bad breath out is to use natural methods. The natural remedies and cures are less likely to cause negative side effects, and cost a lot less. The process of removing your bad breath can be relatively simple once you know the reason behind why it happens.

If there isn't any underlying causes for the bad breath, you are able to use these ways to prevent or treat your breath problem.

Keep your mouth moist

Make sure you keep your mouth wet mouth by regularly hydrating your. Consuming 8 glasses of water per daily is essential to maintain your body's cells' nutrition to perform the functions they are designed to perform. If you aren't able to bring water with you then you could eat candy or chew gum for a boost in saliva production.

The microbes that thrive in moist environments However, the accumulation of microbes and their multiplicity inside your mouth is halted by swallowing occasionally. It is therefore essential to ensure that your mouth is moist constantly to aid in swallowing, and to prevent drying.

Make sure you maintain a healthy oral hygiene

It is an essential routine to be aware of. It is recommended to clean your teeth twice each day. You should brush your teeth daily in order to get rid of food particles that are stuck the spaces between your teeth. It is suggested to use mouthwashes if they do not dry out your mouth. Mouthwashes can reduce bacteria within your mouth. However, certain types can cause dryness which can lead to bad breath.

The mouth is a bed of bacterial growth because it's moist and warm. Therefore, it is essential to maintain your hygiene on a regular basis in order to avoid the development of bacteria. It is essential to clean your teeth properly for maintaining your dental hygiene. The correct way to brush is described in Chapter 5.

Make sure to rinse your mouth with vinegar or soda water to ensure the balance of pH in the mouth.

In the case of excessive acidity Gargling your mouth with soda water can lower the acidity in the mouth. Your mouth is moderately acidic, and an increase in acidity may also interfere with your body's function. The pH in your mouth must be kept at a fragile balance to avoid having bad breath. If your mouth is alkaline, try gargling using vinegar to cause it to become slightly acidic. The pH must be kept at a constant level of 4.5 to 5, so that bad breath doesn't happen.

Consume your meals and eat breakfast.

Many people skip their breakfasts intentionally. Many people are unaware it's breakfast that's the primary breakfast throughout every day. Breakfast is your fuel source throughout your day. A healthy breakfast can also prepare your body in the morning to speed up the process of metabolism of the food you consume throughout the day. If your metabolism isn't as fast then you'll be able to store the fat and calories that are in your body.

If you're on a strict diet then the meal you should not skip is the evening meal since you're not putting in an effort in the evening. Any extra calories consumed at dinner are stored as fat. It is important to have smaller portions of food regularly. Do not eat too much because it will make you sick and not actually shed weight. In fact, you'll increase the chance of developing bad breath.

If you have breakfast for breakfast, you won't have to suffer from acidity as there are food particles that your stomach can digest.

Stay clear of anxiety and stress.

Halitosis is a result of stress and anxiety. It is due to the fact these mood states cause a variety of physiologic reactions that cause imbalances in the body. If you're stressed out or nervous, you'll hyperventilate and cause alkalosis. The blood's acidity and the alkalinity (pH) is altered and disrupts the balance of your body. The disruption can increase the chance of developing bad breath since the pH normal to the mouth can be somewhat acidic.

If you've ever noticed, the lips dry when you're anxious. It's your body's reaction to the stimuli of anxiety and stress. Relax through practicing relaxation methods. Relaxation techniques needn't be complicated. simple breathing exercises that are deep will aid.

Exercise in the standing or sitting or seated. Put your hands on your hips. Inhale with your nose deeply. As you breathe, lift your feet and then stand on your feet. Breathe deeply with your mouth and then lower your heels. Make a mental note to yourself that you should ease into the position. It is also possible to make it sound louder If you can. It is possible to repeat this many times until you are relaxed.

It's a reason for bad breath that's frequently overlooked and left to fend for itself. The majority of people will spend money buying the mouthwashes, mints and deodorizers, but do not know the truth about this. Keep calm and relaxed so that you are less likely to have bad breath.

Consume a balanced and healthy diet

You must eat well-balanced meals for getting rid of smelly breath. An appropriate diet will comprise of sufficient carbohydrate in order that will give your body with energy. If you're physically active throughout your day, boost your intake of carbs However, ensure that you are burning off the calories are consumed. If they don't, they'll remain in the form of fats.

The average person who engages in daily tasks typically burns around 1,800 to 2200 calories for women, while 2,400-3,000 calories for males. The amount of energy required will vary depending on the type of activity an individual performs throughout the daily routine. There are numerous websites that offer calorie calculators are able to calculate how many calories are in food consumed.

Proteins are essential for your body. You need proteins as the building blocks for cell division inside your body. Additionally, your body needs mineral and vitamins for proper bodily function. They are usually found in the fruits and vegetables.

These are approximate percentages of food items that a typical human needs.

Carbohydrate = 45% to 50%

Fats = 20% to 25%

Proteins = 10% to 15%

Minerals and vitamins = between 5% and 10 percent

Consume more vegetables and fruits.

This is due to the importance of this food. Many fruits and veggies contain antioxidants, fibers, chlorophyll and minerals as well as vitamins. All of these are necessary for preventing Halitosis. They can also reduce the stomach's acidity through their alkaline nature. They also provide vital vitamins and minerals that are essential that are essential for body functioning. When your body's functioning well it is the least likely to happen.

Do not take drugs if you are addicted.

Alcohol, tobacco, and other drugs may cause bad breath. This is discussed in Chapter 1. The research has shown that these substances cause dental problems and gum disease. One example of this is smoking cigarettes and tobacco. Smoking cigarettes doesn't just cause a stain on your fingers, it also discolors the lips and teeth, and creates a smell in your mouth. Get rid of smoking cigarettes and experience fresh breath as well as an overall healthier body.

Methamphetamine is an illegal substance that damages the teeth of your body. Barbiturates, cocaine, and opiates are illegal drugs that cause addiction and can be harmful for your overall health. They can cause organ dysfunction including the brain. The same effects are triggered by alcohol. The body is destroyed and cause health problems. Unhealthy bodies emit unhealthy smells that come from the nose and mouth.

Beware of foods that are aromatic

The strong-smelling food items like onion and garlic could create bad breath. So, if your diet includes such foods be sure to clean your teeth immediately after eating. Ingestion of too many spiced condiments are also thought to trigger bad breath. Chewing gum or chewing mints may mask the smell but it's not going to get rid of it entirely. Consuming a lot of water will remove the spiciness.

Maintain a healthy and balanced life style

Healthy living will improve the health of your body and improve its overall wellbeing. When your body's in good health then it emits only pure, fresh smells. A person who is unhealthy will emit smells that are unpleasant and rotten. Avoid allowing it to affect your body. This can be prevented through a healthy diet, sleeping enough drinking water, exercising often, and abstaining from drinking cigarettes, alcohol as well as other drugs.

Chapter 12: Five Natural Remedies to Fight Bad Breath

Prior to the invention of toothpaste and toothbrushes used, herbal remedies and plants were used as cleansing substances for mouths. This list contains proven herbal remedies and plants to prevent bad breath.

Guava

Guava leaves are utilized in the past by people who wanted to eliminate bad breath. If you're unable to find the items you need to clean your mouth and there is no store nearby, you could chew on leaves of guava to freshen up your breath. You can chew on the leaves until you notice the difference. Your breath will smell clean and fresh.

Additionally, you can use the branches to eliminate food or plaque off your teeth. You can cut a small twig to expose the inside. It will function as a toothpick. Make sure not to damage the gums.

Honey

Make a honey-based solution by mixing a teaspoon of honey that is pure and one glass of water. Utilize this mixture to clean your mouth every time you're able. Honey is a great drink for well-being. Honey is known to treat a variety of respiratory diseases due to its antimicrobial properties. Additionally, it is believed to boost the body's immune system.

Green tea

Take a cup of green tea every day to ease dryness in your mouth. This will help to remove food and microbe leftovers. Tea is also a great way to soothe painful throat or bleeding gums. Green tea can be a great drink for relaxation since it's got theanine which has an euphoric effect. As you relax then your breath will be expected to be pleasant, too.

Ginger

While ginger is considered an opulent food item however, it is also antimicrobial that kills bacteria. The ginger is crushed and then cooked until the juice is taken out. Inhale this solution. Allow it to remain for about a minute inside your mouth, to eliminate the bacteria. Rinse using water to get rid of the smell of ginger.

Lemongrass

Lemongrass is used for many purposes in the respiratory and digestive system. Cleanse the lemongrass well before bringing it to the boil. Then let it simmer until the volume of water has been diminished to half the amount. Consume the fluid. It assists in metabolism and digestion, and assists in maintaining the body's health. It's also an antibacterial as well as an aspirin. This will in turn aid in preventing bad breath.

The plants and herbs can be excellent ingredients to treat bad breath as they happen naturally. The natural products are more affordable and safer to utilize within the body. But, be aware that none of the herbs or plants are able to protect you against bacteria or bad breath in the absence of following all steps mentioned in preceding sections.

Chapter 13: A Proper Hygiene Routine

It is crucial to brush properly for maintaining good oral health as well as helping to prevent bad breath. There are times when you're in a rush, and you're certain that the mouthwash you use removes any smell left. It's not true. It is important to know the proper way to brush in order to eliminate foodstuffs that remain in your mouth. Here are some steps to making sure you brush properly.

Step One - Cleanse your toothbrush well prior to using

It's recommended that you store your toothbrush inside the fridge to stop the growth of bacteria. However, before you do this it is essential to clean it clean of any toothpaste or dirt. It is also possible to prepare your toothbrush by boiling it first, and then store it in a spot that is clean. Clean it well before you use it once more.

Make use of a head or toothbrush at a minimum of one month. Purchase a new brush every month to ensure that your bristles remain firm. Choose a brush that has finer bristles in order to avoid damaging the gums.

Step 2 - Clean your molars and side teeth

By using a firm stroke apply a gentle stroke to the teeth on both sides. Use a moving back and forth that is followed by upward and downward strokes. Be sure to perform the same for the interiors as well as the top of your teeth on the sides. Each stroke should be for at least 20 times or more, until you can feel that all food particles have been removed out of your teeth.

Step #3 - Make sure you brush your teeth on the front

Make the same strokes on your front teeth, sideways as well as up and down. It is possible to use additional toothpaste if you need to. The strokes should be repeated minimum of 20 times until the food particles have been eliminated. Your strokes must be strong but not overly hard so as to avoid damage to the gums or teeth.

Step 4 - Clean your gums

Cleanse your mouth before you rinse it and using gentle strokes, brush your gums across your teeth. It is possible to wash your toothbrush, and then use a the latest toothpaste. Make sure you don't damage the gums. Check your tongue to see if you have any leftover gums with food-related patches.

Step 5 - Clean the surface of your mouth, as well as the tongue area

Then, you should brush the areas twenty times, using the horizontal, vertical and diagonal strokes. Look with your tongue any area with food-based coatings. Pay attention to these areas.

Step #6 - Cleanse your tongue along the inside of your mouth

Use a toothbrush to clean your tongue. You can also brush the inside of your tongue also. If you notice a coating of food particles on your tongue, you can use the sterile cotton buds to clean them. It is also possible to get bad breath by the growth of bacteria in your tongue. Therefore, you should brush your tongue horizontally and vertically for at least 20 minutes.

The portion that is the most inner to your tongue close to the throat can be a delicate region, so you should just use your tooth as far as you are able to without vomiting. The tongue is a perfect location for the growth of bacteria which is a the cause of bad breath.

Step 7 - Cleanse your mouth

Cleanse your mouth to make it your mouth is clean. If your teeth are sensitive then you should utilize warm salt water to wash your mouth. Make sure you rinse your throat, too, by moving your chin and taking a sip. Make sure to do this at least 10 times.

Step #8: Floss between your teeth

Cleanse your teeth by flossing them, making sure there are no food particles that get between your teeth get eliminated. The floss should be placed between your gums and the teeth. Microbes are rapidly multiplying within this region due to its moisture and warmth.

Step #9 - Rinse using mouthwash

Gargle with the natural mouthwash, which doesn't result in dry mouth. If you feel it is necessary, dilute the mouthwash by adding water.

Chapter 14: Ten Key Tips on Bad Breath Problems

In order to get rid of bad breath, you need follow the guidelines in the earlier chapters. For those who want to stress or add important points, below are some tips to keep in mind.

The primary reason behind bad breath is a poor state of overall health. If every part that comprise your body well-maintained the bad breath will go away. That includes, obviously the health of your mouth. Unwell bodies emit the "sick" smell.

Balance or homeostasis is an vital element in maintaining healthy health. When your body is in a position to regulate its own homeostasis levels and balance, it is possible to maintain your health. This implies that all elements in your body must to stay within their natural amounts.

Anything that causes dry mouth leads to bad breath. Make sure your mouth is moist at all time.

Find out if you have a pathologic condition first. Before you are able to use organic methods to get rid of bad breath, it is important identify the root of the issue. The natural remedies will work in the event that you are seriously sick.

Get the assistance from a trustworthy friend or family member. If you're unsure whether your breath smell is gone, then seek out a trustworthy friend or family member to assist you get it checked. Naturally, he or will have to sniff your mouth to determine if you suffer from bad breath. However, it's the best way to discover the real truth.

Do not kiss people who have coughs or colds. Infections of the respiratory tract can be passed via the mouth, so avoid being too lavish when it comes to kisses. In addition, many sexually transmitted illnesses are passed on by kissing, so you should be aware. Be forewarned and you will be protected.

Don't put things in your mouth. There is a chance that you have the unwelcome habit of throwing things into your mouth or chewing on things that your hands grab. Beware of this bad habit, as there are a lot of microorganisms. There is a chance that you're introducing bad bacteria to your mouth which could create bad breath. Also, it is recommended to clean your hands prior to eating.

Mouthwashes aren't going to eliminate bad breath if do not address the cause. Eliminating the root of the issue first and then you'll be able to be able to effectively eliminate bad breath.

If you are still suffering from bad breath with an instrument. If there is no one you can trust to detect your breath, it is possible to use the test with a spoon. This can be done by inserting a spoon into the mouth and allow it to remain there for about a moment. Then, you can use it as a lick so that your saliva gets covered with the spoon. Then, take it off and allow it to dry for a short time. Then, take a sniff. If you notice a smell, it's still bad breath.

If at first you don't succeed, don't give up. Try again. There's a chance you've overlooked some thing. The bad breath will not disappear this quickly. It's like washing away the smell of food items that have stuck to your clothes, you'll need to clean often.

Chapter 15: Do You REALLY Have Bad Breath?

Okay, I'm aware that I mentioned we would not be talking about the definition of bad breath however I believe it's important to talk about your options regarding whether you suffer from bad breath.

There's a lot of people that believe they smell bad, but they don't. prior to reading the remainder of this guide and figure out the best way to get rid of the smell of bad breath, try a couple of things to find out if actually do have bad breath!

1) Breathe On The Back of Your Hand

One of the best ways to find out if are smelling bad This is most likely the most straightforward (and perhaps the most reliable). Some people fall into the trap of breathing in your palm The problem with that the smell emanating from it is likely take over the smell of the breath.

When you breathe in the palm of your hand and smell it, you'll be able to detect the smell as it flows out of your mouth. This can give you an picture of what it is that your breath smells like.

2) The Licking Test

Most people are unaware that saliva is scented also and it could affect the way you breath. To determine how saliva smells, take a lick of the back of your hands after which you should wait a while and sniff the area which you've took a lick.

If you can smell it immediately there'll appear to be some odor however, if you wait for just a couple of seconds after you feel the smell, it should fade disappear. If it is gone then you're good take it off, but if it persists, it suggests that saliva may be the source for your breath odor.

3) Check Your Teeth

Take the time to look closely at your smile to determine the presence of any black spots. These black marks on your teeth can be an indication of bad breath. the bad breath that you experience in these cases is often due to gum and tooth issues.

In this moment, you ought to know the likelihood that you are a bit breathy. If not, good luck for you!

If you're similar to the majority of us and do suffer from bad breath, you need to be educated about the issue and find out what the potential reasons for bad breath might be.

It's what we'll be talking about in the following chapter.

Do all three breath tests to determine the truth about whether or not you suffer from bad breath.

Chapter 16: Causes of Bad Breath

Now, it is time to be aware of if you've got bad breath. If so, we'll examine what's the cause! There is no way to figure out the best way to treat it when you don't understand why it's happening initially.

In the meantime, before we go deep into this, it's essential to understand that there are numerous factors that could cause bad breath. But most likely will occur as one of the 10 following things.

1) The Food You Eat

As you may think, it's likely that the food you consume could be the cause of the bad breath you have, but how do you know?

If you eat food, the particles of food remain inside the mouth... even when you can't actually notice or feel the particles, they're present. Everybody knows that foods such as garlic and onions can are a source of bad breath. However, even when you consume odorless food items, it could still produce an unpleasant smell if particles stay in the mouth for excessively long.

2) Dental Issues

Unhygienic dental habits can cause dental problems that could cause bad breath. There aren't many dental problems that don't result in bad breath. Therefore, should you experience any dental problems whatsoever, this is probably the cause of the smell of bad breath.

Dental problems are triggered by improperly brushing your teeth and also by flossing too often.

3) Dry Mouth

When your mouth gets dry this can lead to bad breath. The mouth's interior must always be damp. This is due to the fact that saliva cleanses your mouth. If you don't have saliva flowing through the oral cavity, dead tissue will accumulate on your tongue, which can cause bad breath.

4) Chronic Diseases

Abscesses and oral infections can create a smell that is unpleasant when you chew. A kidney failure can be the cause of this kind of odor.

This kind of smell generally a fishy smell However, the best part is that it disappears once it has a few days.

5) Nose/Throat Infection

Most people aren't aware that allergies can result in bad breath as they often result in the nasal discharge. Once the discharge is at the back of your throat, it'll trickle downwards, which can cause bad breath.

6) Tobacco

If smoking cigarettes, you don't be interested in hearing this, however smoking cigarettes is almost always the cause of bad breath. There are a myriad of reasons behind that, and the primary one is that it can result in your mouth becoming dry. Also, it increases the chance of developing a disease that may create bad breath (like that we have already talked about).

7) Extreme Dieting

In the other direction of the spectrum, smoking cigarettes can be a problem for certain people who are seeking to maintain their health and go to extreme diets. It's not healthy for either your breath or body!

It is due to the fact that when you are on a strict diet, your body can be diagnosed with ketoacidosis. This causes some chemicals to breakdown that cause bad breath.

8) Milk

I love milk! If I could have the entire day, I'd however, some people may be lactose intolerance, and if this is you, then milk could produce bad breath.

9) Alcohol

Alcohol can cause problems with your digestive system and cause your breath to become poor, but it may create dry mouth, which as we all know, can cause bad breath.

10) Stress

Everyone has to deal with, however little people realize that it can result in bad breath. It is due to the fact that when you're feeling stressed the stress can affect the digestive system, which could result in bad breath.

There's no doubt that there are many other issues that could cause bad breath however there's the chance that some of the problems listed can be responsible for the bad breath.

Go through the entire list of the potential issues which could be the cause of the bad breath in your mouth and then determine whether any of them could be a possibility.

Chapter 17: Oral Hygiene (The Proper Way)

From here on, each chapter will be a comprehensive look at how to use science-based methods to eliminate bad breath. It's recommended to try each of these strategies in the course of time, but be sure that you do not get overwhelmed.

One of the primary reason why people don't get rid of their breath issues is due to the fact that they feel overwhelmed by the amount of information available. If you are certain you're doing something is all that's important and you'll be able to get rid of bad breath much faster than you ever thought was possible.

Oral Hygiene is Likely All You Need!

And I am sure you're considering "But I already have proper oral hygiene!"

It's true that it could be, but you're probably going to find there isn't.

The typical American has adequate dental hygiene. It's not that they aren't taking care of their teeth. But the issue is that many people are taking care of their teeth too much! In reality doing too much with your dental oral hygiene may make the situation more difficult.

The Three Key Areas

When we talk about their oral health in the context of oral hygiene, they're talking about three important areas.

1.) The teeth

2.) The gums

3) The Tongue

If you take good charge of the three aspects chances are there's a chance that bad breath could be gone.

We'll discuss ways you can properly care for the three.

1) Brush Twice Per Day

A few people do their dental hygiene once a each day. This isn't enough. People who brush their teeth every meal, which is a lot.

It is important to clean your teeth when you awake and prior to going to sleep.

2.) Cleanse your teeth once every each day

Many people do not floss. But you are able to find people who floss several times each day. If you are flossing multiple times every day, you're harming the gums. It's essential to only floss once a every day. If you do not floss, you let bacteria accumulate even when you brush your teeth.

3) Brush Your Tongue

Yes, it is a bit odd, but little people actually clean their tongue after brushing their teeth.

It is essential to get back in the direction you get without vomiting. The reason this is vital is that not just are food particles accumulating in the mouth however dead cells also build in the tongue, too. This could cause an unpleasant odor.

4) Use a Brush With Small Bristles

It's likely that you didn't know this, but there's an excellent chance that the bristles of your tooth brush aren't enough! The bristles must be tiny enough to be able to reach places which bristles of larger sizes aren't.

5) Replace Your Toothbrush

When it comes to toothbrushes, it's vital that you change your toothbrush every each 12 weeks. After 12 weeks, they diminish in effectiveness.

6) Make Regular Dentist Visits

I am not a fan of the dentist yet I understand how crucial the check-ups are. The need to go to your dentist at least twice a year in order to get an extensive cleaning of the teeth.

If you don't brush or floss each day however the reality is that dental professionals use tools we do not have to can give your mouth a thorough cleaning.

7) Use A Water Pick After You Eat (Optional)

This is totally optional and I've witnessed this make a huge difference to the breath of people. It is not necessary to floss or clean at every meal however there's no harm in making use of a waterpick since it doesn't cause any harm to gums.

8) Drink A Lot of Water!

Anyone who said that 8 glasses of drinking water a day was sufficient is lying! The consumption of 8 glasses water every day is not enough to properly provide the necessary hydration for most people. And the consequences of not being properly hydrated? Dry mouth, and causes bad breath!

Get plenty of water in order so that your mouth does not become dry and dry. If you do notice your mouth getting dry, drink some sips to make it more moist.

9) Start Gargling

If you're not already a gargling syringe this is the perfect right time to get started. As you rest, bacterial may infiltrate your mouth. If you do take a gargle every 30 seconds at the morning and wash your mouth after you're done, you'll be getting rid of any bacteria which could cause an unpleasant smell.

The process of getting rid of bad breath starts with proper dental hygiene. Look over the 9 items listed and ask you, what are your dental hygiene? A majority of us have the basics in place, like flossing and brushing. However, I'm not aware of many people who can actually do each of the nine tasks consistently.

The task for this portion is to stay aware of the nine things and incorporate them throughout your day.

Chapter 18: Let's Break Down The Food You Are Eating

As with most of us, I am a huge foodie and I would love to just sit and say that what you eat aren't affecting your breath however, that they can.

Certain foods can be a complete threat to your breath. The fact is that in order to get rid of your bad breath, then you'll have to eliminate these items.

A diet packed with fats or with sugar can produce bad breath.

The reason is that certain foods are known to cause digestive problems and people with issues in digestion may have bad breath.

Below are some points to consider in relation to your food choices.

* Vegetables and fruits with antioxidants should be consumed. The green leaf,

broccoli as well as berries and cabbage all are great. They can maintain your digestive system in good shape.

* Yogurt which is sugar-free is great to consume because it will assist in keeping away bacteria responsible for creating persistent bad breath.

• Cut down on beverages that contain sugar. This can lead to bacteria to accumulate at the back of your throat.

It is obvious that you need to avoid garlic and onions if aren't wanting your breath to be a stench that evening. But, they won't result in persistent bad breath.

Tea and coffee can be consumed, but they could create a bad smell in your mouth. Be aware that caffeine dehydrates the body so if you are drinking tea or coffee be sure to take plenty of water in order to avoid dry mouth. One reason why we think it is okay to drink is due to the fact that a few research has shown they help fight the bacteria which causes bad breath.

As we're on the subject of food, we can also look at certain minerals and vitamins and their effects on the smell of your breath.

You should up the amount of zinc that you consume, because if aren't getting enough zinc in your diet, it may (and likely will) cause bad breath.

It's great news that it is easy to have a capsule of zinc that contains 60mg every day without having to think about making changes to your diet.

* Insufficient Vitamin B can also lead to bad breath if only consume one Vitamin B6 tablet daily which will aid.

• Try to consume approximately the 6,000 mg of Vitamin C every day. Vitamin C will help remove some built in mucus that causes bad breath.

Look over your food habits and determine which of the principles discussed in this section. Buy zinc Vitamin B, as well as Vitamin C supplements to use regularly.

Chapter 19: Improving Your Digestive System

There has been extensively about your digestive system up until now, and this chapter will be brief and concise due to the fact that most of the treatments we've talked about in the past assist with digestion.

As a brief summary the digestive system could produce bad breath if it isn't functioning correctly. One of the best ways to enhance your digestive system is to pay attention to the food you consume. Here are some suggestions that you can begin doing now to improve your digestion system.

1) High Fiber Diet

It is well-known that fiber aids in digestion, however only a small percentage of us actually consume sufficient fiber. It is recommended to eat whole grains, fruit, as well as vegetables on a regular on a regular basis.

2) It's All About The Enzymes

In the absence of enough enzymes, your digestion system will not function effectively. There's a good thing is that it's easy to take enzyme tablets in each dose.

3) Get Rid of Constipation

We don't like to talk about constipation, however when you're suffering from constipation, it is important to consult your physician as this can create unpleasant breath. A few things that you may attempt to remedy constipation include drinking as well as water.

It could have felt as a recap, since it wasn't. Be sure to be taking in plenty of fiber as well as taking enzymes every meal, and your digestion is healthy.

Chapter 20: Herbal Remedies That Actually Work

There's always a debate taking place about the use of natural cures. One side other side, there are the people who say that the use of herbal remedies can solve any problem and that's the only thing you'll ever require.

At the opposite end of the spectrum, you'll find people who say that herbal treatments are useless and won't assist people out.

It's a mystery why people are discussing this issue, when we have numerous scientific studies that show that the real truth lies somewhere between. While herbal remedies can't fix every problem, they are able to assist with a few things which is great for those who use them. Luckily, among those is bad breath.

In this article, I'll discuss some of the herbs that have been tested to treat bad breath. Do not try all of them simultaneously. If you try a single one, and you find it helpful, then stay with the one that doesn't aid them to move on to the next.

1) Gargling Honey and Cinnamon Powder

Yes, it sounds a little weird does it not? However, it does work! I've actually tried this by myself and have noticed that I've got better air quality throughout the day.

The first thing you should do is to take a few teaspoons of cinnamon powder and honey mixed with warm water. I do this nearly every single day now, and I believe it keeps my breath fresh throughout the every day no matter the food I consume. Does it offer a permanent solution? Not really, but it's still an excellent temporary solution.

2) Chewing Sage

It is another well-known herbal treatment. What's cool about Sage is that it is antibacterial which can aid in getting rid of the smell that is so unpleasant.

3) Using Tea Tree Oil

Tea Tree oil has an component that helps to clean your mouth. It is great at getting rid of harmful bacteria.

It's good to know that toothpaste is now made that contains tea tree oil it. This means that you do not need to purchase tea tree oil to the side. You can easily find toothpaste that contains tea tree oil already.

It isn't necessary to test each of these herbs, however I strongly suggest starting by trying at the very least one. If I were forced to pick the one I'd prefer the combination of cinnamon and honey. Try it this morning to see if it performs!

Chapter 21: Breath Spray...Does it Work?

The topic of breath sprays is a complex topic. Because of this, I believe it should be discussed about in this book.

This is the time to kick with a note that I wouldn't suggest spraying your breath to people...Not suggesting it isn't effective However, the reason I do not recommend the spray is because it can't really solve the issue; it's just a temporarily relief for a couple of minutes.

However, so that you are aware of it being only a temporary covering up, and you're doing it in a way that is geared towards covering up Feel free to use it!

It is important to be mindful when picking the correct air freshener and ensure that it doesn't contain any alcohol. The reason is that at the end of the day alcohol is actually a factor in making the breath smell worse.

It is important to choose an oil-based product and not alcohol-based. Particularly, you'll want it to have peppermint or eucalyptus oils.

It is important to take note that regardless of whether it makes your breath smell lighter, it will not fully cover it Don't go around being convinced that you've got great-smelling breath for the next couple of minutes.

Determine if the breath-spray is something that you wish to purchase. If yes, ensure you purchase one that doesn't contain alcohol, but is rather made of oil.

Chapter 22: Over The Counter Medications

Okay, let's tackle the myth of now...over prescription medications DO NOT work!

Certain, prescription medicines will help you get rid of the smell of bad breath, however you're not likely to have success using over-the-counter medications.

Some of you are considering "but I have tried them in the past and they worked". That's awesome and truthfully, they may have been successful However, those that perform best are those which contain the herbs that are natural within them, which we spoke about in a couple of chapters back.

If you bought these herb at an MUCH lower cost than when that of the OTC drug, you'd be getting the same results.

Now How About We Talk About What Does Work...

This is included under the OTC medicines section, because while it's technically not a medicine, it's available in any shop and will improve the bad breath you have.

And what exactly am I discussing on this particular occasion?

Flaxseed!

This is vital to those with bad breath. Actually, Flaxseed can do more than any OTC drug would.

The reason why it performs very well is that it is a rich source of Omega-3. Omega-3 is a fat acid which helps fight the effects of fat breath.

Simply sprinkle flaxseed into your cereal or in your yogurt. You will not even notice it.

Do not waste your hard-earned cash for Over The Counter Medication! Instead, purchase flaxseed, and sprinkle it on the food you eat.

Chapter 23: Show Me The Quick Remedies! !

This is the part that gets fun The quick solutions to get rid of your bad breath. When you're looking through these solutions, keep in mind that they are not all provide a permanent solution. They may provide an interim solution and can be utilized to get your breath to smell nice for a short period of time.

If, for instance, you're going out on the night with a partner, you should use one or two of these methods to make sure your breath smells nice throughout the entire evening.

Now let's dive straight into it, and then examine some quick solutions.

1) Drink Water

It has been discussed several times in the past and drinking water is the best methods to ensure that you don't have unpleasant breath throughout the day. The more dry your mouth becomes, the more bad your breath will be a stench.

2) Have Some Gum

It is certainly one of the fastest methods to get your breath fresher However, be aware that there are some who find it offensive to chew their gum in the front of others and if you do this, the breath you'll likely be back to the way it was prior to that.

3) Rinse Your Mouth

Every morning and at night you should wash your mouth immediately after you've cleaned your teeth.

4) Scrape Your Tongue

So long as you scrub your teeth as well as scrape your tongue prior to going out, you won't need to fret about breath for another few days. You'll be amazed by the extent to which scraping your tongue will aid in removing bad breath.

5) Use Parsley

Personally, I'm not fond of chewing gum. I've never had and likely never ever. So, I use parsley in place of. If you chew parsley for just a few minutes before washing your mouth, it will refresh your breath for several hours.

These are, however, short-term fixes that should only be employed in situations of emergency. In reality, there are a lot of solutions that work for the short-term that you can use, however I have listed these five options because they're the best for everyday normal living. If you find yourself experiencing an emergency and require fresh breath, you can use any of these five options.

Chapter 24: Let's Just Prevent It...Shall We?

Okay, we're at the chapter that is most significant in the entire book.

We offered you many great suggestions for removing bad breath. However, now we're at the stage where we must be discussing ways to eliminate permanently the smell and the best way to keep it from ever returning after it's gone.

As we mentioned earlier the lack of dental hygiene is the primary cause of bad breath. And if they were to fix it, the bad breath will go out of their mouths.

One of the chapters is actually devoted to oral hygiene. However, let's discuss it in greater detail because this will the most effective treatment.

Flossing

YOU MUST FLOSS! If you don't floss, you're likely to develop bad breath. Bad breath and flossing are inextricably linked.

Flossing can reach areas that the toothbrush cannot reach and if you're not getting the areas, then the bacteria build-up and your breath can begin to be stale.

A common mistake is that they brush their teeth first and after flossing. This is actually reversed. The first step is to floss, and the second is to scrub your teeth.

There's lots of argument regarding what kind of floss to choose and which is better than another, but the fact is, it doesn't really matter much. Unwaxed or waxed, Super thing, or long and super flavor or not It doesn't matter.

It is important using floss to cleanse the area of your teeth which your brush is not able to remove.

Brushing

If people think of their oral health the first thing they consider is cleaning. They believe that the more often they brush, the more clean their mouth is going to be. But that's not the reality. When you clean your teeth more than two times per day, it's more harmful than positive.

With that being said now, let's discuss the initial step in correct brushing, which is to choose the proper brush.

If you want to buy the 45-degree toothbrush but the best part is that most of them are 45 degrees however you must ensure that you check prior to purchasing.

Also, we mentioned that you must purchase toothpaste that contains tea tree oil. Although this isn't a necessity, however, it will assist in getting rid of the bacteria responsible for bad breath.

After you've finished cleaning your teeth, you haven't completely finished your brushing!

It is imperative to brush your tongue If you do not want to smell bad. Actually, as it comes to eliminating bad breath it could be even more essential as brushing your teeth (although this isn't a reason to cease the habit of brushing the teeth).

If you'd like to go this step further, and do not want to make use of your toothbrush in order for your tongue brush You can purchase the tongue scraper which is actually more efficient. In the meantime, your toothbrush should suffice.

If you floss at least once a day and brush twice every day, clean your tongue immediately after brushing your teeth, then clean your mouth after you're done. Over the course of time, your breath will be better.

When your breath is "normal" again, all you need to keep up with these routines so that the smell won't come back.

Develop a routine of the hygiene practices we covered in this section. For a short period of time, performing this routine every day, and bad breath will disappear. Avoid the mistake of trying this one time and abandoning because you did not notice any results. Try the process for 30 consecutive days and you'll be amazed at the difference in how the breath will smell after 30 days.

Chapter 25: The Vulgar Affector of Halitosis Halitosis

If you've been rushing into marriage, and your spouse is Jew and you'd like to find to know more, here's an answer to Find out if your spouse is a bit sour and you should break up with her. In a book called Talmud in which Jewish law and traditions are built on, bad breath is believed to be a major handicap and any husband who figures that his wife is suffering from this condition could be able to terminate the ketuba, also known as the marriage contract.

Bad breath, a condition also referred to as halitosis is an extremely serious problem that is affecting 35 to 45 percent of people and does more than affect their relationship. Even though a severe instance can snuff out the flames of love Bad breath is not just an indication of a lack of dental hygiene, but also an indication of other illnesses and conditions including Sjogren's syndrome, diabetes chronic bronchitis or xerostomia as well as other.

A solution to unpleasant breath in a hurry is imperative not due to the social ill-feeling the issue causes, but due to the fact that due to the fact that it's primarily caused due to periodontal diseases caused due to poor oral hygiene it's linked with coronary artery disease (commonly known as heart disease) that kills about 600,000 individuals in the United States every year. Interestingly, however, doctors are now beginning to realize the benefits of maintaining the best dental health in order to prevent heart attacks There is a better method to evaluate the health of our mouths than by taking a few breath.

Your Bad Breath can Kill Your Heart

If a person fails to follow the correct oral hygiene routine, such including flossing and brushing the oral bacteria that are normally found within the mouth multiply and feed off food particles in between the teeth, in plaques inside the gums, as well as in the tongue's coating. of your tongue. In the process of consuming leftover food particles as well as decaying cells inside the mouth bacterial generate a gas with a smell that is the most common cause of the unpleasant breath.

Researchers have speculated that at a specific moment in the course of an infection with periodontal bacteria, the bacterium in the gums and mouth are introduced into bloodstreams, which sets off an immune reaction like inflammation. Researchers believe that regardless of the presence or absence of an infection, inflammation can increase the risk of forming blood clots. Clots can decrease blood flow towards the heart, which results in there is a lack of oxygen. It is then forced to strain to compensate for this deficiency, thereby raising blood pressure, and increasing the likelihood of having a heart attacks.

Disadvantages of Having a Bad Breath

As the way you dress will reveal more about your character, so too can the smell of your breath. According to the American Dental Association (ADA) estimates that over 80 million people living in the US are suffering from persistent Halitosis (persistent smell of bad breath). While it's not as common that it affects one out of four Americans and greatly affecting sufferers in so many ways that they shell out more than 10 billion dollars each year in dental hygiene products to treat the condition.

Below are some of the disadvantages of having halitosis

A bad breath can ruin any opportunity to have a relationship. Because the majority of intimate relationships involve kissing, having a bad breath can make the process difficult to enjoy. A persistent and frequent bad breath can deter a person from engaging in a romantic relationship. It is proven by an online survey by Match.com with 5,000 singles in who 2,150 of them identified fresh breath as the primary factor to consider before agreeing to dating and ranked dental halitosis in the top three characteristics that make a person look unattractive to the person you are looking to marry. People with bad breath are often found to have fewer chances of meeting potential partners, go out more often, and lesser chances of getting engaged.

The smell of bad breath can lower self-esteem. If sufferers notice those who are avoiding conversations about their breath or making snide remarks regarding the smell of their breaths, a decline in self-esteem will follow in a predictable manner. It could cause anxiety as well as depression and stress. It may cause difficulties with friends as well as romantic relationships. It could also cause a decline in productivity at work and in school and ultimately leads to further depressing the self-esteem of sufferers.

A bad breath-related condition is associated with low earnings. The study shows that people with chronic halitosis are more likely to be part of the class of people who earn lower and are less likely to be promoted. The reason for this is that bad breath can negatively impact your image and also your career prospects. According to the Australian Breath Clinic warns that as job opportunities become more competitive and employers becoming more specific, employees in customer service, or that interact with customers are likely to be dismissed when they fail to comply with a stringent set of standards, which includes one that assures them of good breath.

Three kinds of Odors that are associated with Breath Problems

The smell of mouth that is halitosis-related can be classified into three types based upon the quality of their odor:

www.ingramcontent.com/pod-product-compliance
Lightning Source LLC
Chambersburg PA
CBHW062138020426
42335CB00013B/1256